The Chemotherapy R[ecipe Book]

250+ Quick and Easy Breakfast, Lunch, Dinner, Dessert and Snack Recipes [for Those]
Undergoing Chemotherapy

Minute Help Guides

Minute Help Press
www.minutehelp.com

© 2012. All Rights Reserved.

Table of Contents

DISCLAIMER 7

HOW TO BOOST CHEMOTHERAPY WITH NUTRITION 8

BREAKFAST RECIPES 10
- Honey Oatmeal 11
- Apple and Pear Oatmeal 12
- Buttermilk Pancakes topped with Fruit 13
- Cinnamon Raisin French toast 14
- Apple Cinnamon Quinoa Bran 15
- Blueberry Oat Bran Muffins 16
- Strawberry Oat Bran Muffins 17
- Pear Bran Muffins 18
- Fruit Filled Egg Crepes 19
- Vegan Crepes 20
- Zucchini Egg Bake 21
- Quick Egg Omelet with Tomatoes 22
- Scrambled Egg Sandwich 23
- Veggie Egg Sandwich 24
- Tofu Omelet 25
- Breakfast Bagel 26
- Canadian Bacon Bagel 27
- Honey & Apricot Breakfast Bread 28
- Pumpkin Loaf 29
- Berry Bread Loaf 30
- Fried Egg on Toast 31
- 3 Minute Herb & Mushroom English Muffins 32
- Four-grain Porridge Mix 33
- Buttermilk Waffles 34
- Quick Grits 35
- Mushroom & Rice Frittata 36
- Wheat-Germ Buttermilk Pancakes 37
- Tomato Basil Quiche 38
- Baked Garlic Cheese Grits 39
- Apple Breakfast Bread 40
- Banana French Toast 41
- Banana Fritters 42
- French Toast Topped with Spice Pears 43
- Breakfast Potato Patties 44
- Sweet Barley Bowl 45
- Fruity Breakfast Smoothie 46
- Sautéed Fruit Wraps 47
- Green Berry Breakfast Smoothie 48
- Banana Chocolate Spelt Muffins 49
- Raisin-Rice Pudding 50
- Homemade Nutty Granola 51
- Grilled Pineapple/Mango and Yogurt 52
- Sesame Porridge with Dried Fruit 53
- Homemade Trail Mix and Yogurt 54
- Tangy Citrus Breakfast Shake 55
- Poached Apricots and Bagels 56
- Nutty Quinoa with Coconut Milk 57
- Sweet Potatoes with Raw Honey 58
- Whole Wheat Bagels topped with Fruit 59

    Morning Fruit Fritters 60
LUNCH RECIPES **62**
    Broccoli Soup 63
    Tuscan Tomato Soup 64
    Mushroom Pea Soup 65
    Cauliflower Soup 66
    Mushroom Broth 67
    3 Minute Simple Gazpacho 68
    Vegetarian Chili 69
    Squashed Pizza 70
    Barley and Dilled Chicken Salad 71
    Whole-Grain Veggie Pizza 72
    Broccoli and Red Peppers 73
    Chicken, Broccoli and Veggies 74
    Chinese Cabbage Sauté 75
    Turkey Marsala 76
    Mexican Red Snapper 77
    Fish Fillets Sandwich with Tomato Relish 78
    Summer Roasted Vegetables 79
    Indian Aloo Phujia 80
    Indian Lamb Tagine 81
    Quick Chicken Korma 82
    Portuguese Stew with Kale 83
    Bean, Mushroom and Couscous Salad 84
    Mediterranean Chopped Salad 85
    Spicy White Bean Salad 86
    Cauliflower Broccoli Salad 87
    Cranberry Salad 88
    Spicy Broccoli Pasta 89
    Asian Style Pasta 90
    Cannery Row Soup 91
    Comforting Minestrone Soup 92
    Spicy Bar-b-cue Chicken 93
    Chicken Ratatouille 94
    Turkey Stuffed Cabbage 95
    Easy Zucchini Parmesan 96
    Penne Pasta Classic 97
    Broccoli Soup 98
    Spicy Miso Soup 99
    Wild Rice Gourmet Salad 100
    Sausage Stuffed Mushrooms 101
    White Chicken Chili 102
    Roasted Veggie Salsa 103
    Split Pea Soup 104
    Tomato Soup 105
    Baked Dijon Salmon 106
    Marrakesh Vegetable Curry 108
    Quick and Light Asparagus Soup 109
    Thai Butternut Soup 110
    Loaded Baked Potato 111
    Mediterranean Chickpea Salad 112
    Mango Salsa Patties 113
DINNER RECIPES **114**
    Stuffed Chicken Breasts 115
    Butternut Squash Curry 116
    Lamb Shanks with Mushrooms and Cauliflower 117

Spaghetti Casserole	118
Stewed Beef Dumplings	119
Baked Pineapple Rice Casserole	121
Easy Lentil Carrot Stew	122
Alphabet Soup	123
Sablefish with Bok Choy	124
Caponato	125
Easy Potato-Cheese Casserole	126
Irish Corn Beef & Cabbage	127
Slow Cook Beef & Cabbage	128
Greek Stew	129
Garlic Mashed Potatoes	130
Spicy Vegetable Rice	131
Indian Butter Chicken	132
Fajita Pizza	133
Grilled Trout	134
Rice Kabsa	135
Quick Vegetarian Dinner Wrap	136
Stove-Top Stuffed Potatoes	137
Chicken Curry in Tomato Puree	138
Campfire Salmon Fillets	139
Indian Chicken Do Pyaaza	140
Indian Fish Fillets	141
Spicy Red Corn Chowder	142
Stuffed Baked Tomatoes	143
Vegetable Biryani	144
Rava Dosa	145
Salmon Lemon Bake	146
Mediterranean Pasta and Shrimp	147
Mushroom Garlic Pasta	148
Halibut with lemon egg sauce	149
Quick Mediterranean Dinner Wraps	150
Spinach Bowl with Olives and Pine Nuts	151
Mushroom Ciabatta	152
Seafood with Pasta Casserole	153
Greek Oven Bake	154
Chicken Snow Peas with Pasta	155
Indian Butter Chicken	156
Mediterranean Roasted Fennel with, Feta, Prawns and olives on Pasta	157
Mediterranean Chicken Pasta	158
Honey Soy Broiled Salmon	159
Orzo with Olives and Feta	160
Greek Beef & Peas	161
Lean Pork Chops over Rice	162
Crockpot Pork Roast Dinner	163
Chinese Barbecue Spareribs	164
Chicken with Panang Curry	165
Tofu and Basil over Brown Rice	166
Alfredo Italian Sausage Casserole	167
Vegan Jambalaya Oyster	168
Chicken Veggie Curry Casserole	169
Tofu Ginger & Garlic	170
Green Gazpacho	171
Egyptian Lentil Soup	172
Garlic Soup	173
Fish Soup & Wild Rice	174
Pasta Checca	175
Roasted Comforting Vegetables	176

- Chakchouka – Moroccan Cooked Tomatoes & Peppers 177
- Sweet Crumbed Chicken 178
- Shrimp & Okra Gumbo 179
- Fast Mango Fish 180
- Beef Massaman Curry 181
- Sour-Creamed Meatballs 182
- Chicken in Tempura Batter 183
- Fried Green Garlic Tomatoes 184
- Zucchini & Veggie Hash Browns 185
- Easy Broccoli and Cauliflower With Cheese Sauce 186
- Quinoa Soup with Avocado and Corn 187
- Bulgur Salad topped with Tuna, Olives and Feta 188
- Wild Rice and Turkey Salad w/ fruit 189
- Smoked Trout with yogurt dressed Pasta 190

SNACKS 191

- True Blue Smoothie 192
- Banana Nut Milkshake 193
- Choco Smoothie 194
- Tropical Smoothie 195
- Beach Blonde Smoothie 196
- Mango Lime Smoothie 197
- Pumpkin Protein Smoothie 198
- Homemade Granola with Yogurt 199
- Pear & Raspberry Crumble 200
- Banana Raspberry Soft Serve 201
- Quick Crepes 202
- Apricot Balls 203
- Sesame Honey Snack Bars 204
- Sweet Potato Pudding 205
- Banana Nut Cookies 206
- Fruit on-a-stick 207
- Nutty Maple Oaties 208
- Berry Choco-Muffins 209
- Vanilla Custard 210
- Old Indian Comfort Pudding 211
- Hot Fruit Compote 212
- Ginger Brown Snack Bread 213
- Sticky Sugared Nuts 214
- Spooned Peaches 215
- Caramel Apples 216

DESSERT RECIPES 217

- Single Surprise Chocolate Chip Cake 218
- Love in a Cup - Red Velvet Dessert 219
- Comforting Corn Pudding 220
- Coffee-Creamed Brownies 221
- Mediterranean Citrus & Olive Oil Cake 222
- Berry Cake 223
- Apple Crock Pot Betty 224
- Soft Carrot Pudding 224
- Banana Nut Cake 225
- Banana Spice Cake 226
- Raspberry Pudding Cake 227
- Apple-berry Yogurt Parfait 228
- Peanut Butter Candy Log 229
- Fabulous Fudge 230
- Banana Milkshake 231

CREAM PUFFS 232
QUICK PINEAPPLE ORANGE GELATIN DESSERT 233
APPLE PUDDING MUFFINS 234
ORANGE DREAM MOUSSE 235
LOVELY LEMON SORBET 236
AFTER DINNER FRUIT & DIP 237
PEAR AND APPLE COMPOTE 238
COCONUT ALMOND MACAROONS 239
NATURAL PEANUT BUTTER COOKIES 240
FRUIT PARFAIT DELIGHT 241

ABOUT MINUTE HELP PRESS 244

Disclaimer

The following recipes were collected and written with careful research; they were not, however, prepared by an oncologist. The recipes that follow are meant to help and give ideas to someone undergoing chemotherapy. Before starting any diet, you should always consult your doctor.

How to Boost Chemotherapy with Nutrition

The medicines used to treat cancer during chemotherapy include a large assortment of various drugs. Unfortunately, all the benefits of chemotherapy will come at a cost. The disease and its treatments will alter the cancer patient's immune system, lowering the body's natural defenses. While some chemo drugs are cell-specific, seeking out damaged and mutated human cells to slow down and kill, there are other drug combinations that will also kill-off healthy cells. Yet, there are ways to stimulate a cancer patient's natural immune system to help battle the disease, and stimulate antibodies while working in unison with chemotherapy treatments to make the drugs more effective.

There are many natural whole foods that support the chemotherapy cancer patient. While antioxidant therapy is controversial, supporting chemotherapy treatments with a strong dietary regimen can reduce the negative effects of chemo and improve your chances for achieving the best possible outcome.

Research studies have proven that proper nutrition will enable the body to better handle the stress of multiple drugs and provide the patient with more energy. Over the years we have become more scientific and holistic in our approach to treating cancer. Whereas past generations believed you would eat to speed recovery, scientists now understand the correlation between good nutrition and healing.

Nutrition has been linked to cancer in many different ways. There has been research done to show that certain food choices may cause cancer or prevent it, and some foods have been shown to drastically decrease the risk of it reoccurring. However, there are certain foods that can negatively affect the benefits of chemotherapy, thus limiting a cancer patient's treatment.

Before any group of food hits the store shelves, manufacturers spray, inject and append these items to minimize any bacterial growths, as well as preserve the food for a longer shelf life. This strategy can be dangerous to cancer patients because of unnecessary toxins conflicting with a suppressed immune system. This problem can be alleviated by using whole, all-natural and organic foods whenever possible.

Additionally, cancer patients must avoid food items that have the potential of enduring bacterial contamination. For example, avoid salad bars, sushi bars, raw or undercooked meat, fish, shellfish, and eggs, when at all possible. By following safe food practices, chemotherapy patients and their caregivers can eliminate risking any food-borne illnesses.

- Before consuming, wash fruits and vegetables thoroughly.
- Cook foods to proper temperatures in order to eradicate any bacteria; meat, poultry, and seafood should be well cooked.
- Foods must be stored promptly, at low temperatures to minimize bacterial growth (below 40°F).

Another concern for chemotherapy patients is the amount of sugary products and the effect it has on cancerous cells. The German biologist, Otto Warburg, discovered that malignant tumors are dependent upon glucose consumption. In other words, cancerous cells feed on the sugar we consume.

When we eat sugar or white flour products, the blood glucose levels rapidly rise. The body immediately releases doses of insulin that enable glucose to enter the cells. In short, the sugar stimulates cell growth and thus, acts as fertilizer for tumors.

Chemotherapy patients clearly must adopt a lifestyle change and overhaul the daily menu. The way we choose our food, the ingredients in our list of options and the overall method of how we eat can make a huge difference in the battle with cancer.

Breakfast Recipes

The notion of going on a cancer diet can be daunting. Just the thought of it brings to mind bland, unappetizing meals.
Not so! You can eat very well and never sacrifice flavor, while helping your immune system tolerate chemotherapy and boosting the effects of your medicines. Try starting your day with these delicious breakfast recipes.

Honey Oatmeal

2 cups skim milk
1 ½ cups of distilled water
1 teaspoon ground cinnamon
1 cup of old fashioned rolled oats

¼ cup of wheat germ
¼ cup of almonds
3 tablespoons of raw honey

Directions:
Place milk, water, and cinnamon in a saucepan and bring to a boil. Stir in the oats and wheat germ and return to a boil. Reduce heat to low and cook, stirring until thickened for about 5 to 8 minutes. Stir in almonds and top with natural raw honey.

Apple and Pear Oatmeal

1 cup rolled oats

1 cup skim milk

1 cup water

1 apple and 1 pear, chopped

¼ teaspoon cinnamon

¼ teaspoon of nutmeg

Directions:

Place the rolled oats, water and skim milk into a pan on low heat. While stirring, simmer for approximately 5 minutes. While the oatmeal is simmering, mix in fruit, cinnamon and nutmeg and stir.

Buttermilk Pancakes topped with Fruit

2 cups whole wheat flour
1 tablespoon baking powder
2 teaspoons of raw honey
2 organic eggs

2 tablespoons canola oil
1 ½ teaspoons vanilla extract
1 cup of mixed berries (strawberries, raspberries, blueberries)

Directions:
Combine flour, baking powder and raw honey in a bowl. In another bowl, whisk together the buttermilk, eggs, oil and vanilla. Combine the mixtures and whisk until smooth. Heat a nonstick griddle or regular frying pan over medium heat. Spoon approximately 1/3 cup of batter into the pan or griddle. When one side is done, you'll begin to see bubbles appear on top, about 2-3 minutes.
Flip pancakes over with a spatula and cook for another minute. Transfer to plate and repeat process with remaining batter. Top with fresh fruit.

Cinnamon Raisin French toast

2 eggs
2 egg whites
3/4 cup skim milk
½ teaspoon vanilla extract
½ teaspoon ground cinnamon

3 slices cinnamon raisin bread
2 teaspoons unsalted butter
1 tablespoon maple syrup
2 tablespoons water

Directions:
Whisk the eggs, egg whites, skim milk, vanilla extract, and cinnamon in a medium bowl. Pour into a shallow pan. Arrange bread slices in the pan and press gently to help them soak up the liquid, flip over to other side so that both sides are coated.
Coat a skillet with unsalted butter and place over medium heat. When the skillet is hot, place bread into pan and let brown; flip over to other side and allow to brown. Remove bread from pan and drizzle with syrup.

Apple Cinnamon Quinoa Bran

1 apple, medium-sized, peeled and chopped (best to use McIntosh or Gala)

1 cup distilled water

1 cup of Quinoa, rinsed and drained

1 teaspoon wheat germ

1 teaspoon of flax seed

½ teaspoon agave syrup

1 teaspoon almonds, slivered

½ teaspoon cinnamon

Directions:

In a medium-sized pot bring 1 cup of distilled water to boil. Add in quinoa slowly and reduce heat to medium; add in agave syrup and continue stirring constantly to thicken. Remove pot from heat; proceed to add the chopped apples, wheat germ, and the flax seed. Top with the slivered almonds and sprinkle cinnamon on top.

Blueberry Oat Bran Muffins

2 cups oat bran

¼ cup agave syrup or diabetic blueberry jams

2 teaspoons baking powder

1/4 teaspoon baking soda

1/2 cup low-fat vanilla yogurt

1/2 cup orange juice

2 organic eggs

2 tablespoons olive oil

3/4 cup fresh blueberries

Directions:
Combine the oat bran, syrup or jam, baking soda, and baking powder in a large bowl, and mix well. Combine the orange juice, vanilla yogurt, fresh blueberries, eggs and olive oil in a bowl and stir. Add both mixtures together and stir well.

Use nonstick cooking spray to coat the bottom of muffin cups, and then fill 3/4 of the way with the mixture. Bake at 350F for about 15 minutes. Test with a toothpick, inserted in the center of the muffin to make sure it comes out clean. When done, allow to cool thoroughly before removing from muffin cups.

Strawberry Oat Bran Muffins

2 cups oat bran

¼ cup diabetic strawberry jams

2 teaspoons baking powder

1/4 teaspoon baking soda

1/2 cup low-fat vanilla yogurt

1/2 cup orange juice

2 organic eggs

2 tablespoons olive oil

3/4 cup fresh strawberries

Directions:
Combine the oat bran, strawberry jam, baking soda, and baking powder in a large bowl, and mix well. Combine the orange juice, vanilla yogurt, fresh strawberries, eggs and olive oil in a bowl and stir. Add both mixtures together and stir well.
Use nonstick cooking spray to coat the bottom of muffin cups, and then fill 3/4 of the way with the mixture. Bake at 350F for about 15 minutes. Test with a toothpick, inserted in the center of the muffin to make sure it comes out clean. When done, allow to cool thoroughly before removing from muffin cups.

Pear Bran Muffins

1 1/4 cups of low fat buttermilk

2 large eggs, lightly beaten

1 1/4 tablespoons cinnamon

1/4 teaspoon salt

1 1/2 teaspoons vanilla extract

3 tablespoons canola oil

1 medium pear, cut into small slices

1 1/4 teaspoons baking soda

1 oz agave juice or 2 tablespoons SPLENDA substitute for baking

1 cup wheat bran

1 1/2 cups whole grain wheat flour

Directions:
Combine the whole grain wheat flour, wheat bran, SPLENDA, cinnamon, baking soda, and salt in a large bowl. In a separate bowl, combine the two large eggs, low fat buttermilk, canola oil, pears, and vanilla extract.

Combine all ingredients together and mix well. Pour batter into muffin cups and bake for approximately 15 to 20 minutes. Allow muffins to cool completely before removing from muffin cups.

Fruit Filled Egg Crepes

2 tablespoons heavy cream

2 large organic eggs

1 tablespoon canola oil

½ cup of fresh berries

Directions:

Whisk heavy cream and eggs together in a bowl. Heat a pan with canola oil on medium heat. Pour the mixture into the pan and allow eggs to slowly cook. When crepes begin to separate themselves away from the edges of cooking pan, carefully turn them over.

Slide the finished crepe onto a plate and top with fresh fruit.

Vegan Crepes

½ cup almond soy milk

½ cup distilled water

1/4 cup coconut oil

2 tablespoon raw honey

2 tablespoons maple syrup

1 cup buckwheat flour

Directions:

Blend distilled water, almond milk, coconut oil, raw honey, maple syrup, and buckwheat flour. Place covered mixture in fridge for 1 hour to chill.

Take a small pan and grease lightly with coconut oil. Heat pan on medium heat then ladle batter onto pan. When crepe has a golden hue, gently flip to other side. Serve with yogurt.

Zucchini Egg Bake

1/2 cup skim milk

3/4 cup egg beaters

½ teaspoon of parsley

1 teaspoon pepper

1 teaspoon thyme

2 tablespoons of chopped garlic

1 small onion, chopped

2 medium sized zucchini, grated

Directions:
Spray a large pan with cooking spray and sauté zucchini, onion, garlic, parsley, and thyme until al dente or when they feel tender, yet crisp. This will take approximately 10 minutes. Remove from the heat and let cool.

Set the oven to 350F. In a bowl, combine egg substitute, skim milk, and hot sauce and mix well. Add egg mixture to vegetable zucchini mix and blend well. Next, pour mixture into casserole dish then place in oven and bake for 35 minutes until eggs have puffed and set together.

Quick Egg Omelet with Tomatoes

6 large egg whites

2 medium whole tomatoes

Dash of pepper

Directions:
Fry three egg whites and use a Teflon pan that won't require any oil. While the eggs are cooking, chop up two medium-sized tomatoes. Once egg whites have been cooked, top with tomatoes and season with pepper.

Scrambled Egg Sandwich

Olive Oil cooking spray

1 organic egg

Finely chopped chives

2 slices whole grain bread

Spreadable light cream cheese

Directions:
Heat a frying pan on moderately low heat; lightly coat pan with olive oil cooking spray. Whisk egg, and add in chopped chives; pour into pan and gently stir until scrambled. Toast the whole grain bread, spread a little cream cheese onto bread, and then place egg onto sandwich.

Veggie Egg Sandwich

Olive Oil cooking spray

1 organic egg

Finely chopped chives

2 thinly sliced tomatoes

1 teaspoon white onion, chopped

2 slices whole grain bread

Spreadable light cream cheese

Directions:
Heat a frying pan on moderately low heat; lightly coat pan with olive oil cooking spray. Whisk egg, chives and onion; pour into pan and gently stir until scrambled. Toast the whole grain bread and spread with a little cream cheese. Spoon scrambled egg mixture onto sandwich and top with 2 thinly sliced tomatoes.

Tofu Omelet

1 cup tofu

1/4 cup rice milk

2 tablespoons coconut oil

1 Portobello mushroom, sliced

1 shallot, finely chopped

1 cup Parmesan cheese

2 tablespoons chopped parsley

2 slices whole grain bread

Directions:

Crumble tofu into rice milk; add sliced mushroom and shallot. Pour coconut oil in a frying pan on medium heat. Pour tofu mixture into pan and stir until soft and blended.

Sprinkle omelet with parsley and parmesan cheese. Serve with side of toasted whole grain bread, or top bread with it scrambled and eat it as an on-the-go sandwich.

Breakfast Bagel

1 plain whole grain bagel

1 tablespoon soft Alouette (can also use cream cheese)

½ cup mixed greens

3 slices of Roma tomatoes, thinly sliced

½ cup chopped green onions

½ cup fresh berries

Directions:

Split a whole grain bagel and lightly toast. Spread a good helping of alouette, only on one side of bagel, then top with greens, sliced Roma tomatoes and diced scallions. Serve with a side of various berries (strawberry, raspberry, blueberries).

Canadian Bacon Bagel

1 plain whole grain bagel

2 slices Canadian bacon, chopped

½ cup grated parmesan cheese

3 slices of Roma tomatoes, thinly sliced

½ cup chopped basil

¼ Green Pepper, sliced

3 button top mushrooms

2 tablespoons canola oil

Directions:

Heat oil in a small nonstick pan over medium heat; add Canadian bacon and cook on each side. Add green pepper to pan and mushrooms to pan and sauté.

Split a whole grain bagel and lightly toast. Top with cooked bacon, mushrooms, sliced Roma tomatoes and green peppers and sprinkle basil and parmesan on top.

Honey & Apricot Breakfast Bread

2½ cups soy flour

1½ cups whole wheat flour

¼ cup sunflower seeds and flax seeds

1 packet of dried yeast

2 teaspoons ground cinnamon

1 teaspoon salt

1½ cups skim milk

¼ cup raw honey

1/4 cup chopped dried apricots

¼ cup unsalted butter, melted

Directions:

Sift flour together in a large bowl. Stir in sunflower seeds, flax seeds, yeast, ground cinnamon and salt. Next, form a well in the center of mixture.

Combine raw honey and low fat milk. Stir continuously over a low heat. Add the liquid mixture to the dry flour ingredients, stirring to form blended soft dough.

Dough should be moved to a lightly floured surface, then knead for about 10 minutes. The dough should be smooth and stretchy. Place stretchy dough in a bowl that has been lightly greased, and set aside in a warm, dark place and cover with towel. Dough should sit until it has risen and doubled in size.

Preheat oven to approximately 350°F. Lightly grease a pan to place dough into.

Place dough onto a lightly floured surface and knead for 2-3 minutes. Roll out to a rectangle that depicts a bread loaf. Sprinkle the apricots over. Place the dough on tray and generously brush butter over it. Bake for 30 minutes. Transfer to a wire rack to cool.

Pumpkin Loaf

¼ cup coconut oil

2 tablespoons thyme

2 cups soy flour

½ teaspoon baking soda

½ teaspoon salt

½ teaspoon ground nutmeg

½ teaspoon cumin

½ cup SPLENDA sugar substitute

1 cup mashed pumpkin

½ cup skim milk

1/3 cup canola oil

Olive oil cooking spray

2 organic eggs

Directions:

Melt coconut oil in a pan over medium heat. Mix soy flour, baking soda, salt, cumin, thyme and nutmeg in a bowl. Stir in SPLENDA sugar.

In a separate bowl, combine pumpkin, skim milk, oil and eggs. Combine all ingredients together and mix well; Preheat oven to moderate, 300°F and lightly coat a loaf pan with olive oil cooking spray. Spoon pumpkin mixture into loaf pan and bake approximately 1 hour. Allow to cool in pan 10 minutes, and then transfer to a wire rack to cool completely.

Berry Bread Loaf

¼ cup butter

2 cups soy flour

½ teaspoon baking soda

½ teaspoon salt

½ teaspoon ground cinnamon

½ cup SPLENDA sugar substitute

½ cup raspberries

½ cup strawberries

½ cup skim milk

1/3 cup canola oil

Olive oil cooking spray

2 organic eggs

Directions:

Melt butter in a small pan on medium heat.

Mix soy flour, baking soda, salt, and cinnamon in a bowl. Stir in SPLENDA sugar substitute.

In a separate bowl, combine raspberries, strawberries, skim milk, oil and eggs. Combine all ingredients together and mix well; Preheat oven to moderate, 300°F and lightly coat a loaf pan with olive oil cooking spray. Spoon berry mixture into loaf pan and bake approximately 1 hour. Allow to cool in pan 10 minutes, and then transfer to a wire rack to cool completely.

Fried Egg on Toast

2 slices whole grain bread
2 tablespoons unsalted butter
2 large organic eggs

1 teaspoon grated parmesan shavings
Black pepper

Directions:

Heat a frying pan on moderately low heat; lightly coat pan with olive oil cooking spray. Whisk egg, pour into pan and allow frying; flipping over once to allow other side to lightly brown and set. Toast the whole grain bread and then place egg onto sandwich. Sprinkle grated parmesan shavings over fried egg and toast. Serve with a side of warm ginger tea with raw honey.

3 Minute Herb & Mushroom English Muffins

4 shitake mushrooms, trimmed
1 tablespoon extra virgin olive oil
1 teaspoon chives
1 teaspoon of tarragon leaves

1 fresh lemon, juiced
1 garlic clove, minced
1 teaspoon chopped parsley

Directions:

Combine minced garlic, parsley, chives, tarragon leaves and lemon juice. Place shitake mushrooms on toast, then top with herb and lemon mixture. Finish by sprinkling extra virgin olive oil over the mixture.

Four-grain Porridge Mix

½ cup millet grits

½ cup coarse bulgur

½ cup untoasted kasha

½ cup barley flakes

1 ½ cups raisins

1 tablespoon cinnamon

1 teaspoon nutmeg

Combine millet, bulgur, buckwheat, barley flakes, raisins, cinnamon and nutmeg in a bowl and blend to create a porridge mix.

Buttermilk Waffles

1 large organic egg
1 cup buttermilk
3 tablespoons safflower oil
2 tablespoons raw honey
1 cup whole-grain flour

1 tablespoons baking powder
1 teaspoon baking soda
1 teaspoon cinnamon
Olive oil spray for waffle iron
Raw honey or fresh fruit

Directions:

Combine lightly beaten egg, buttermilk, oil and honey in a bowl. Stir in whole grain flour, baking soda, baking powder and cinnamon.

Lightly spray waffle iron with olive oil cooking spray to cover grid. Heat the waffle iron and add batter. Remove when waffle is set. Top with raw honey and/or fresh fruit.

Quick Grits

1 cup of soy milk
2 teaspoons raw honey
1 pinch salt

1/4 cup quick cooking grits
2 tablespoons of fresh cranberries

Directions:

Combine soy milk, honey, and salt and bring to a boil over high heat. Slowly stir in grits, allow boiling, and then reducing heat to low. Cover and cook slow, stirring occasionally to avoid lumps. Allow grits to thicken, about 3 to 4 minutes.

Let stand for 1 minute. Garnish with a few cranberries.

Mushroom & Rice Frittata

2 cups water to boil wild rice
1/2 cup wild rice
1 teaspoon salt, for wild rice
5 large organic eggs
2 large egg whites
2 tablespoons parsley, chopped
1/2 teaspoons salt, divided
1/2 teaspoons ground pepper
1/4 teaspoons nutmeg
2 teaspoons extra-virgin olive oil
1 cup chopped red onion
1 tablespoon minced rosemary
2 cups of mushrooms shiitake sliced
1/2 cup finely shredded Parmesan cheese

Directions:

Wild rice preparation: Bring 2 cups of water to a boil; add wild rice and teaspoon of salt. Cover, reduce heat and allow rice to simmer for about 45 minutes, until the rice is tender. Drain water off.

Frittata: After you have began cooking the rice, whisk eggs and egg whites in a bowl, then combine with parsley, salt, pepper, and nutmeg. Preheat broiler.

Heat the olive oil in a deep skillet or a cast-iron pan, over medium heat. Add the chopped red onion and pepper; cook, stirring, until softened, about 3 minutes. Next, toss in shitake mushrooms; stir frequently and cook until liquid has been absorbed, about 6 minutes. Reduce heat to a medium setting; next, stir in the rice and rosemary.

Take the rest of egg mixture and pour evenly over rice and vegetables. Cover partially and cook until the egg sets, about 5 to 10 minutes. Top with Parmesan cheese. Pan should be placed under broiler until the eggs are fluffy and the top is browned, about 3 minutes. Let stand before serving.

Wheat-Germ Buttermilk Pancakes

1 cup whole wheat flour

1/2 cup wheat germ

1/4 cup SPLENDA sugar substitute

1 teaspoon baking powder

1/2 teaspoon baking soda

1/4 teaspoon salt

Cooking olive oil spray

1 1/4 cups buttermilk

1/4 cup canola oil

2 large organic eggs (separated)

2 cups fresh fruit (bananas, berries, or raisins)

2 cups low-fat vanilla yogurt

Topping: 2 cups fresh blueberries

Directions:

Combine the whole wheat flour, SPLENDA, baking powder, baking soda, wheat germ, and salt. In a separate bowl, mix the egg yolks, buttermilk, and canola oil. Egg whites should be beaten lightly until they form stiff peaks.

Lightly spray griddle with olive oil and heat over medium-low heat; spoon 1/3-cup portions of batter onto the griddle. Reduce the heat to medium-low. Cook until you see tiny bubbles appear on top of pancakes, then turn over and cook for a couple minutes more.

Spread yogurt and fresh blueberries over the top of pancakes.

Tomato Basil Quiche

1 tablespoon extra virgin olive oil

1 onion, diced

2 Roma tomatoes, half peeled and half sliced

2 tablespoons soy flour

2 teaspoons dried basil

3 organic eggs, beaten

1/2 cup low fat milk

Salt and pepper

1 unbaked pie crust – 9 in deep dish

1 1/2 cups Colby-Monterey Jack cheese, shredded

Directions:

Preheat oven to 400 degrees. Place pie shell in oven for 5 minutes to brown.

Heat olive oil on a medium setting. Sauté onion until soft; and remove from skillet. Lightly flour tomato slices and sprinkle with basil, then sauté 1 minute on each side. In a small bowl, whisk the eggs and low fat milk. Sprinkle lightly with salt and pepper.

Layer 1 cup of shredded Colby-Monterey jack cheese in the bottom, on top of pie crust. Layer the diced onions over the cheese, and top with roma tomatoes, and then pour egg mixture on top. Top with the last of shredded cheese. Bake for 15 to 20 minutes at 350 degrees or until filling is puffed, fluffy and golden brown.

Baked Garlic Cheese Grits

1 cup uncooked grits
4 cups distilled water
1 tablespoon salt
1/2 cup unsalted butter

1/2 lb. sharp cheddar cheese, grated
2 tablespoon Worcestershire sauce
2 teaspoons minced garlic

Directions:
Boil grits in salted water; when grits are done, add remaining ingredients and mix. Pour into lightly greased casserole dish, top with sharp cheddar cheese. Bake in 350 degree oven for 20 minutes.

Apple Breakfast Bread

3 eggs, beaten
2 cups SPLENDA sugar
1 cup canola oil
1 tablespoon vanilla extract
3 cups all-purpose soy flour

1 tablespoon baking soda
1 teaspoon cinnamon
3 to 4 apples, cored and chopped
1 cup chopped pecans

Directions:
Combine fresh eggs, SPLENDA sugar, canola oil and vanilla until well mixed and set aside. In a separate bowl, mix soy flour, baking soda and cinnamon; stir this into egg mixture. Next, place the apples and pecans in the mixture. Divide batter equally between 2 well-greased and floured loaf pans. Bake at 325 degrees for 1 hour, or until breakfast bread is golden

Banana French Toast

3 ripe bananas
3/4 cup hemp milk or almond milk
1-1/2 teaspoons ground cinnamon
1/2 teaspoon pumpkin pie spice

2 teaspoons vanilla extract
6 slices of whole grain bread
2 tablespoons coconut oil

Directions:
Blend bananas, milk, cinnamon, pumpkin pie spice, and vanilla in blender; and pour mixture into dish and then gently dip bread slices into the mix, coating both sides. Fry in coconut oil over a medium-hot skillet until golden brown. Serve with maple syrup, raw honey or top with fruit.

Banana Fritters

3 bananas
½ cup canola oil
1 cup soy flour
2 teaspoons baking powder
¼ teaspoon salt

1 tablespoon SPLENDA sugar
¼ cup heavy cream or soy milk
1 organic egg beaten lightly
½ tablespoon lemon juice

Directions:
Sift dry ingredients together and blend well. Beat egg, add heavy cream or milk and combine. Mash bananas thoroughly and mix with lemon juice; add to egg/cream batter and mix well. Heat oil in skillet on medium heat; drop the batter by tablespoonful's into deep, hot oil. Drain off oil; Sprinkle the powdered sugar on top.

French Toast Topped with Spice Pears

4 tablespoons raw honey

2 teaspoon ground cinnamon

1 teaspoon ground ginger

1 tablespoon lemon juice

2 large pears, peeled and sliced

2 large organic eggs

1/3 cup almond milk

2 slices whole grain bread

1/4 cup toasted sliced almonds

Directions:

Preheat oven to 350 degrees F and lightly oil a baking dish. Blend the raw honey, 1/2 teaspoon cinnamon, and 1/2 teaspoon ginger and the lemon juice together in a small bowl; spread evenly into the bottom of the baking dish. Arrange the sliced pears covering the bottom of the baking dish. Beat the organic eggs, 1 tablespoon raw honey, 1 teaspoon cinnamon, and ground ginger together in a shallow dish; soak each slice of bread in the egg mixture and lay over pears.

Bake in the oven until the bread is golden brown, about 20 minutes. Top French bread with almonds and drizzle with any honey, cinnamon and ginger left over.

Breakfast Potato Patties

2 ounces mashed potatoes
2 ounces bread crumbs
1 ounce coconut oil
1 teaspoon sage

½ teaspoon salt
½ teaspoon pepper
2 eggs
1 cup bread crumbs.

Directions:
Mash potatoes and mix with sage, salt and pepper and ½ cup bread crumbs; blend well together, add the egg, and form a patty; Beat 1 egg and pour into flat dish. Pour ½ cup bread crumbs onto plate. Roll patty in the egg and then dip into bread crumbs, and fry in the one ounce of coconut oil. Place on plate with towel.

Sweet Barley Bowl

1 cup cooked organic barley
1 tablespoon. raisins
1 tablespoon. chopped almonds

½ chopped green apple
½ fresh banana
1 teaspoon pure maple syrup

Directions:
Combine all ingredients in a bowl and mix well. Drizzle with shredded coconut.

Fruity Breakfast Smoothie

10 ounces of organic coconut milk
½ cup frozen berries
½ frozen banana

1 tablespoon. shredded organic coconut
1 tablespoon. dark coco powder

Directions:
Add the coconut milk to the blender; add in frozen berries and frozen banana, Blend well. Add shredded coconut and coco powder and blend well.

Sautéed Fruit Wraps

Whole grain crepes
1 large green apple, chopped into small pieces
½ cup golden raisins
1 banana
2 tablespoons SPLENDA brown sugar
½ teaspoon pumpkin pie spice
Organic Maple syrup

Directions:
Mix the apples, raisins, brown sugar and pumpkin pie spice thoroughly; warm over low heat on the stove. Spoon 2 tablespoons of the mixture into crepes. Fold each crepe over and place several slices of fresh banana on top of each fruit crepe. Top with maple syrup.

Green Berry Breakfast Smoothie

1 cup of organic coconut milk
2 frozen bananas
½ cup of frozen mixed berries

2 teaspoon raw honey
½ cup fresh orange juice
2 cups chopped spinach

Directions:
Add liquid ingredients to your blender first; Add frozen ingredients next and drizzle raw honey on top of frozen berries in the blender. Blend well. Next, add the spinach and blend again. Add more coconut milk until you reach the desired consistency.

Banana Chocolate Spelt Muffins

3 cups of organic spelt flower
2 cups of buttermilk
2 eggs, slightly beaten
½ cup pure maple syrup

2 teaspoons vanilla extract
3 tablespoon melted butter
3/4-cup mini dark chocolate chips
2 mashed ripe bananas

Directions
In a large bowl soak the flour in the buttermilk for 12-24 hours. Mix in the remaining ingredients and
place into muffin tins. Make sure the muffin-tins have been well-oiled. Fill them only ¾ full and bake at 325 degrees for 1 hour or until an inserted toothpick comes out clean.

Raisin-Rice Pudding

1 cup of uncooked whole wheat
½ cup of coconut sugar
1 teaspoon sea salt
5 1/2 cups of almond milk

1 cup of raisins
1 teaspoon cinnamon
1 ½ teaspoon almond extract
Heavy whipping cream

Directions
Mix rice, sugar, almond milk, and salt in the top pan of a double boiler and cover. Simmer the water in the lower boiler. Cook the rice until it is thick, about 2 hours, stir frequently. Stir in the extract and raisins
Add a spoon of fresh whipped cream before serving

Homemade Nutty Granola

1 cup of whole rolled oats
1 cup of jumbo oats
½ cup dried cranberries
¾ cup organic sunflower seeds
1 tablespoon flax seeds

½ cup of slivered toasted almonds
¼ cup sunflower oil
¼ cup of raw honey
½ cup of coconut flakes

Directions:
Heat the oven to 250 degrees. Combine the oats, seeds and nuts in a mixing bowl. Warm the oil and honey in a large saucepan until melted. Take the pan off of the heat and add the dry mixture. Stir well and spread the mixture out evenly over two cookie sheets. Bake until mixture is crisp - for about 45 minutes. To prevent sticking, you'll want to stir every once in a while. Take cookie sheets out of the oven. While granola is hot, stir in the coconut flakes, cranberries, and raisins. Allow granola to fully cool then it can be stored in an airtight container.

Grilled Pineapple/Mango and Yogurt

1 large pineapple
1 large mango
¼ stick margarine
Sprouted bread toasted

Organic plain yogurt
Pure honey
2 teaspoons ground cinnamon
Natural vanilla extract

Directions:
Cut the fresh pineapple into thick wedge pieces. Slice the mango into wedge pieces. Heat the fruit on a griddle pan over medium heat. Brush melted margarine over fruit. Cook for 6 minutes, turning once. Line a pan with foil. Place the fruit on the pan and put under a high broiler for 3 minutes on each side. Toast the sprouted bread. Place the fruit on the bread and top with fresh yogurt drizzled in honey. Add a few drops of pure vanilla and the cinnamon on top.

Sesame Porridge with Dried Fruit

½ cup oat flakes
2 cups almond milk

¾ cup mixed dried fruits
4 tablespoon toasted sesame seeds

Directions:
Place the milk, oats and dried fruit into a non-stick pan. Bring the mixture to a boil and lower the heat.
Simmer gently for 3 minutes, or until thick. Serve with a little almond milk and sprinkle with the sesame seeds.

Homemade Trail Mix and Yogurt

½ cup dried figs
½ cup dried apricots
1/2 cup raw walnut halves
½ cup sunflower seeds

½ cup pumpkin seeds
½ cup coconut flakes
1/2 cup raisins
1/2 cup dried banana pieces

Directions:
Combine all your ingredients and place in an airtight container. Shake up well and serve ½ cup of trail mix on top of fresh organic yogurt.

Tangy Citrus Breakfast Shake

1 pineapple
7 oranges, peeled and chopped
1 tablespoon lemon juice
1 tablespoon lime juice

1 pink grapefruit, peeled and cut into quarters
1 cup of coconut milk

Directions:
Pineapple should be sliced into bite-sized chunks. Place the pineapple, oranges, grapefruit, lemon and lime juices into a food processor or blender and blend until thoroughly mixed. Press the juice through a fine strainer to remove any larger pieces of pulp. Blend the juice again adding a few ice cubes and the coconut milk.

Poached Apricots and Bagels

3 cups of filtered water
½ cup agave nectar
4 strips of organic orange peel

1 pound of ripe apricots cut into quarters
Whole-wheat sprouted bagels

Directions:
Simmer water, agave nectar and orange peel on the stove in a medium saucepan over medium heat.
Add in the apricots and push them down so that the liquid covers them. Cook until the apricots are tender, 5 minutes or so. Toast bagel and serve with warm apricots on top. Drizzle with syrup left in pan.

Nutty Quinoa with Coconut Milk

1 cup quinoa
¼ cup slivered almonds

¼ cup coconut milk

Directions:
Pour quinoa into a strainer and rinse well. Pour quinoa into pot with 2 cups of water. Bring pot to a boil, lower heat and simmer gently for 15 minutes. Take the pan off of the heat and let grain sit for a minute.
Pour into a bowl and sprinkle with almonds and pour coconut milk on top.

Sweet Potatoes with Raw Honey

2 large sweet potatoes Raw honey
Unsalted Butter Pumpkin pie spice

Directions:
Place the sweet potatoes in a pot of water and bring the water to a boil. Boil the potatoes for 15 minutes or until the skin comes off the potato easily. Allow potatoes to cool and remove skin. Mash the potatoes in a bowl with 1 tablespoon of butter and drizzle raw honey over the potatoes and sprinkle with pumpkin pie spice.

Whole Wheat Bagels topped with Fruit

2 Whole-wheat sprouted bagels, split
Handful of Raspberries
Handful of Strawberries
Handful of Blueberries

Directions:

Lightly toast 2 whole wheat bagels and top with fresh berries.

Morning Fruit Fritters

2 Large organic eggs
4 ounces strawberries

4 ounces raspberries
1/3 cup coconut oil

Directions:

Whisk eggs and add in strawberries and raspberries. Heat a skillet with 1/3 cup coconut oil over medium heat. Spoon two portions of mixture into pan and cook on each side for 2 minutes. Fold over.

Lunch Recipes

The best lunches for chemotherapy patients provide lots of nutrient-rich vegetables that keep the body energized and hydrated.

Broccoli Soup

1 bunch broccoli, florets only, chopped

2 small parsnips, peeled and sliced

1 medium onion, minced

1 large celery, thinly sliced

3 cups vegetable broth, low sodium

½ teaspoon ground pepper

½ teaspoon salt

Fresh parsley for garnish

Directions:

Combine the broccoli, parsnips, onion, celery, broth, and pepper in a soup pot over medium heat. Cover and bring to a boil, then lower the heat and simmer until vegetables are tender; about 20 minutes.

Puree soup in a blender until smooth. Serve hot, garnished with parsley.

Tuscan Tomato Soup

6 tablespoons extra virgin olive oil

6 cloves garlic

1 bunch fresh basil

1 ½ cups thinly sliced Italian bread

4 cups fresh tomatoes, or one 28-can ounce

1 small medium dried chile

2 cups warm chicken broth or vegetable broth

Black pepper to taste

Directions:

Place oil, garlic cloves and about 1/3 of the basil leaves in a soup pot, over medium heat. Simmer for several minutes, but do not brown garlic. Remove garlic and set aside for later.

Add the sliced bread to the pan and cook, stirring continuously, for 10 minutes. Allow bread to soak up and absorb flavor of the garlic. Add the tomatoes, chiles and about 1/3 of the basil leaves and the garlic cloves. Lower heat and add ½ cup of the broth, allow simmering for 1 hour. Continue to add the remainder of broth in increments during cooking.

Add remaining 1/3 of basil and then puree the soup in a blender. Add pepper to taste.

Mushroom Pea Soup

3 cups dry split pea

4 cups vegetable broth

2 carrots, diced

2 celery stalks, diced

1 yam, peeled and diced

1 ½ pounds of shitake mushrooms, sliced

1/3 cup miso

1 cup water or broth

Directions:

Combine split peas and vegetable broth in a soup pot and bring to boil over high heat. Lower heat, cover and simmer for 45 minutes, stirring often. Add more broth if the split peas become too dry, but not too much. Soup should be thick.

Add carrots, celery, yams and mushrooms. Cover and simmer about 30 minutes, until split peas are tender and falling apart. All vegetables should be tender. Mix miso with water or broth and then stir into the soup.

Cauliflower Soup

- 1 tablespoon sesame oil
- 1 medium onion, sliced
- 2 cloves garlic, minced
- 2 teaspoons ground coriander
- 2 teaspoons cumin powder
- 1 teaspoon curry powder
- 4 cups vegetable broth or chicken broth
- 2 cups chopped cauliflower
- ½ pound medium tofu, cubed
- 3 tablespoons lemon juice
- 1 teaspoon salt
- 3 tablespoons parsley for garnish

Directions:

Heat oil in a soup pot, over medium heat, then add onions, stirring occasionally for about 10 minutes. Stir in garlic, coriander, cumin and curry powder and continue to cook. Stir for another minute.

Add broth, cauliflower, tofu, lemon juice, and salt. Bring to a boil, then lower heat, cover and simmer for 10 minutes. Once soup has cooled down, proceed to puree in a blender. Garnish with parsley.

Mushroom Broth

2 tablespoons extra virgin olive oil

2 cups sliced fresh shitake mushrooms

2 cups sliced fresh Portobello mushrooms

1 medium shallot, chopped

3 cups water

3 cloves garlic, chopped

1//4 teaspoon salt

¼ teaspoon pepper

Directions:

Put oil in a heavy pan over medium heat. Add mushrooms and sauté for about 20 minutes or until lightly browned. In the last 5 minutes, add the shallots, garlic, salt, and pepper. Add water and bring to a boil. Reduce heat and simmer for 30 minutes.

3 Minute Simple Gazpacho

2 cups chopped tomatoes

1 cup peeled and coarsely chopped cucumber

¼ cup extra virgin olive oil

1/3 cup freshly squeezed lemon juice

½ teaspoon sea salt

½ jalapeno, seeded and minced

1 large garlic clove, chopped

2 cups finely chopped tomatoes

½ red bell pepper, finely chopped

¼ cup finely chopped red onion

½ cup chopped fresh parsley

Directions:

Place ingredients in a food processor and blend until pureed and smooth. You can also use a blender; however, blend a little at a time. Pour soup into a bowl and enjoy right away.

Vegetarian Chili

¼ cup extra virgin olive oil

1 cup chopped celery

2 onions, chopped

1 jalapeno, seeded and minced

1 cup chopped shitake mushrooms

1 medium red bell pepper, chopped

6 cloves garlic, minced

3 tablespoons chili powder

2 ½ tablespoons ground cumin

1 teaspoon ground oregano

Dash cayenne pepper

2 cups cooked pinto beans

2 cups cooked kidney beans

2 cups black beans

Two 8-ounce cans crushed Italian tomatoes

Avocado slices for garnish

Parsley for garnish

Directions:

In a large heavy saucepan warm olive oil, over medium heat. Add celery, red bell pepper and jalapeno and sauté until tender – about 10 minutes. When they are tender, add garlic and onions, stirring occasionally. Slowly add in your various beans, mushrooms, chili powder, cumin, oregano and cayenne pepper and continue to stir. Add in the crushed tomatoes, stir mixture and bring to boil. Reduce heat, cover and simmer for 20 minutes. Garnish your chili with avocado slices.

Squashed Pizza

4 cups grated summer squash

1 ½ cups grated Mozzarella cheese

4 tablespoons egg substitute

½ pound ground lamb

1 medium coarsely chopped onion

1 tablespoon chopped fresh oregano

1 tablespoon chopped fresh basil

1 ½ cups marinara sauce

2 cups cheddar cheese

Directions:

Preheat oven to 425. Combine summer squash, Mozzarella cheese, and egg substitute. Press into a greased pan. Bake this mixture for 20-25 minutes.

In medium sized skillet, brown lamb with chopped onion, oregano and basil, then set aside. Pour marinara sauce over crust, sprinkle with lamb mixture and top with cheddar cheese. Bake for 15 minutes.

Barley and Dilled Chicken Salad

1 cup quick cooked barley

Pinch of sea salt

1 ½ cups grated carrot

½ cup dried currants

¼ cup olive oil

2 cups cooked chicken

3 tablespoons fresh squeezed lemon juice

½ cup dill, chopped

Directions:

In a heavy 2 quart pot, bring 2 ½ cups of water and salt to a boil. Stir in barley. Cover and cook over medium heat until barley is tender – about 10 minutes. Drain off any excess water, spoon onto plate for later.

Combine chicken and grated carrot, currants and fresh dill. Add in olive oil and lemon juice and toss to blend. Spoon over barley.

Whole-Grain Veggie Pizza

1 tablespoons extra-virgin olive oil

Olive Oil cooking spray

1 Whole grain pizza crust

6 Roma tomatoes, roughly chopped

3/4 cup ricotta cheese

1/2 cup shaved Parmesan

1 green pepper, sliced thin

1 red pepper, sliced thin

2 cloves garlic, minced

2 tablespoons fresh rosemary leaves

1/4 cup fresh basil leaves, chopped

Directions:
Preheat oven to 475 degrees. Lightly oil the baking sheets with cooking spray. Place whole-grain crust on baking sheet and brush each with 1 tablespoon olive oil. Top crust with ricotta, sliced tomatoes, sliced peppers, minced garlic, rosemary and basil leaves. Bake crust until lightly browned, 10 to 12 minutes. When done, sprinkle parmesan cheese over top of pizza.

Broccoli and Red Peppers

1 bunch broccoli, cut up into bite sized pieces

2 tablespoons extra virgin olive oil

1 tablespoon coconut oil

2 tablespoons unsalted butter

1 medium sized red bell pepper, sliced into strips

1 clove garlic, minced

2 tablespoons pine nuts

Directions:

In a large pan, sauté broccoli in oil and butter for about 4 minutes. Add bell peppers, garlic and pine nuts. Sauté 2-3 minutes, or until vegetables are al dente.

Chicken, Broccoli and Veggies

1 bunch broccoli, cut up into bite sized pieces

2 boneless, skinless chicken breasts, lightly pounded

2 tablespoons extra virgin olive oil

1 tablespoon coconut oil

2 tablespoons unsalted butter

1 medium sized red bell pepper, sliced into strips

1 cup shitake mushrooms

1 clove garlic, minced

2 tablespoons pine nuts

Directions:

In a large pan, sauté chicken breasts for about 3 min on each side. Remove from pan and slice into strips. Next combine broccoli and chicken in pan and sauté in oil and butter, about 4 minutes. Add bell peppers, mushrooms, garlic and pine nuts. Sauté 2-3 minutes, or until vegetables are al dente.

Chinese Cabbage Sauté

½ head of cabbage

½ teaspoon mustard seed

1 teaspoon cumin seed

1 teaspoon fennel seeds

1 to 2 jalapeno peppers, seeded and diced

¼ cup coconut oil

1 teaspoon turmeric

¼ sea salt

Directions:
Heat skillet over medium heat and add mustard seeds, stirring the seeds. Add cumin and fennel seeds and cook until the seeds begin to pop, about 4 minutes. Watch that they do not burn. Remove from pan and set aside.
Blanche the cabbage in boiling water for about 1 to 2 minutes; then allow cabbage to drain. Heat a large sauté pan over medium heat and add jalapenos peppers. Cook for 1 minute and then add cabbage, allow to cook, stirring often. Add mustard seeds, cumin and fennel seeds, oil, turmeric, and salt and sauté for about 5 minutes.

Turkey Marsala

2 tablespoons extra virgin olive oil

2 boneless turkey breasts, lightly pounded

1 cup shitake mushrooms

1 cup sliced onion

½ cup Marsala wine

½ cup fresh or frozen peas

½ cup sliced carrots

2 tablespoons fresh parsley

Directions:
Heat a large skillet over medium heat. Add 1 tablespoon of olive oil, then add turkey breasts. Cook about 3 minutes each side and remove from skillet. Add remaining oil, mushrooms and onion to skillet; cook and stir about 5 minutes. Reduce heat to low. Add wine, peas and carrots and simmer. Return turkey to skillet and coat with sauce. Top with parsley.

Mexican Red Snapper

1 pound of red snapper
½ teaspoon sea salt
¼ cup fresh lime juice
1 medium yellow onion, thinly sliced
1 medium red bell pepper, thinly sliced

2 cups diced tomatoes
1 4 ounce green chiles, mild and chopped
1 tablespoon capers
½ cup chopped cilantro

Directions:
Wash fish, pat dry and place in a glass oblong bowl. Lightly salt and pour the lime juice evenly over the fillets. Cover and refrigerate for 1 hour.
Sauté onion in a skillet, over medium heat. Allow onions to become tender. Add half of bell peppers and all tomatoes, chiles and capers. Cover and cook for about 10 minutes. Add fish and the other half of bell pepper and cook uncovered for about 5 minutes on each side. Sprinkle cilantro over fish.

Fish Fillets Sandwich with Tomato Relish

2 wholegrain sandwich buns

½ pound fresh white fish fillets, de-boned

Extra virgin olive oil

Sprouts

Lettuce

1 avocado, peeled and sliced

Tomato Relish

½ cup chopped red bell pepper

1 cup chopped onion

2 cloves garlic, minced

1 chopped tomatoes

Juice of 1 whole lemon

1 tablespoon agave nectar

Directions:
Grill fish fillets for about 5-10 minutes. In a bowl, combine all tomato relish ingredients and simmer for about 15 minutes.
Place fillet on wholegrain bun, top with tomato relish

Indian Lamb Tagine

2 pounds lamb stew meat

¼ teaspoon cayenne pepper

1 teaspoon ground cinnamon

2 teaspoons paprika

¼ teaspoon ground turmeric

½ teaspoon ground cardamom

½ teaspoon ground cumin

1 teaspoon sea salt

½ teaspoon ground ginger

¼ teaspoon ground cloves

½ teaspoon saffron

¾ teaspoon garlic powder

¾ teaspoon ground coriander

3 tablespoons extra virgin olive oil

2 medium yellow onions, coarsely diced

5 peeled carrots (cut carrots into fourths and then slice into thin strips)

3 cloves finely minced garlic

1 tablespoon grated ginger

1 whole zested lemon

14 ounces chicken broth (choose homemade or low-sodium canned broth)

1 tablespoon sun-dried tomato paste

1 tablespoon raw honey

Directions:

Place cubed lamb in a bowl and toss with 2 tablespoons of the olive oil; set bowl aside. Blend spices together in a re-sealable bag – paprika, cinnamon, cardamom, saffron, turmeric, cumin, cayenne, cloves, salt, ginger, garlic powder, and the ground coriander; mix well. Add the lamb to the bag and coat by tossing lamb around. Refrigerate at least 8 hours, preferably overnight to marinate.

Use a large heavy pot to heat a tablespoon of olive oil. Next add 1/3 of the cubed lamb, and brown on all sides. Remove from heat and set aside; repeat browning with remaining lamb. Add the yellow onions and sliced carrots and cook for 5 minutes. Stir in the finely minced garlic and ground ginger and continue cooking for an approximately 5 minutes. Place the cubed lamb back into pot and gently stir in the chicken broth, lemon zest, tomato paste, and raw honey. Allow this mixture to first boil, then you'll reduce the heat, cover pot and allow to simmer for 2 hours; stir occasionally until the meat is tender.

You can thicken your dish with cornstarch and water if consistency is too thin, but wait until the last 5 minutes before adding any cornstarch.

Quick Chicken Korma

3 tablespoons extra virgin olive oil

3 tablespoons unsalted butter

2 large yellow onions, coarsely chopped

6 tablespoons unflavored yogurt

2 teaspoons sea salt

2 tablespoons mango chutney

4 teaspoons garlic, finely minced

2 teaspoons ground turmeric powder

2 teaspoons Garam Masala

1 teaspoon chili powder

4 chicken breasts, boneless skinless and chopped

1/3 cup slivered almonds

Directions:

Preheat oven to 350 degrees ; lightly grease a deep baking dish.

Over medium heat, heat the olive oil and unsalted butter in a skillet. Cook onions until soft.

Place yogurt, chopped onions, mango chutney, chili powder, turmeric, garlic, and garam masala into blender and mix until a smooth sauce; consistency should look like a thick cream. If too thin, add more yogurt to thicken. Lay chicken evenly into baking dish; add the yogurt/onion sauce over the chicken.

Bake in oven for 30 minutes at 350 degrees, or until the chicken is cooked. Top lightly with sliced almonds.

Portuguese Stew with Kale

1 bunch kale
2 teaspoons minced onion
1 cup brown rice
2 cups low-sodium chicken broth

1 can diced tomatoes
2 bay leaves
6 ounces chorizo, slice thin
1 16-18 ounce can kidney beans, rinsed

Directions:
Wash kale thoroughly and cut fibrous portion of stem. Cut leaves into ½ inch strips. Set a 6-quart pot over medium heat; add rice to brown for 2-3 minutes. Stir in onion and lightly toast for about 2 minutes. Gradually add broth and 3 cups of water. Stir in tomatoes, bay leaves, chorizo and kidney beans. Cover, bring to boil.

Uncover and add kale (as much as you can fit) into the liquid. Cover and cook until kale begins to wilt. Stir and add any remaining kale. Continue cooking over high heat until all kale is wilted. Turn heat down, stirring occasionally, until kale is tender and rice is fully cooked, about 10 minutes.

Bean, Mushroom and Couscous Salad

2 tablespoons extra-virgin olive oil

1 cup couscous

1 ½ cups distilled water

½ cup button mushrooms, sliced

1 small bunch scallions, thinly sliced

1 1/4 cups fresh corn kernels

1 can (16 ounces) black beans, rinsed and drained

2 tablespoons fresh lime juice

1 jalapeno pepper, thinly sliced

Directions:
In a medium saucepan, over medium heat, heat 1 tablespoon of olive oil. Add couscous and brown lightly, about 3 minutes. Add 1 1/2 cups distilled water and bring to a boil. Cover and reduce heat to low; let simmer allowing liquid to become absorbed and couscous is tender. Rinse all vegetables and pat dry. Chop up vegetables, add to a bowl. Add couscous, black beans, and lime juice, and toss to combine all ingredients.

Mediterranean Chopped Salad

3 tablespoons olive oil

2 teaspoons grainy mustard

Salt and ground pepper

1 small head romaine lettuce, sliced

1/2 cup chopped red peppers

1/2 cup roasted almonds, chopped

1 can (15 ounces) chickpeas, rinsed and drained

1 orange bell pepper, seeded, cut thinly

Directions:

In a small bowl, combine lettuce, chopped red and orange peppers and chickpeas. Whisk together the oil and grainy mustard and pour over the chopped salad. Top with roasted almonds.

Spicy White Bean Salad

2 bunches broccoli florets; stems removed
3 large garlic cloves, thinly sliced
5 teaspoons extra-virgin olive oil
1 cup cherry tomatoes
1 tablespoon chopped fresh oregano
1/4 teaspoon crushed red pepper flakes
1 1/2 teaspoons Dijon mustard
1 teaspoon fresh lemon juice
2 cups canned and drained large white beans
2 cups baby spinach

Directions:

Whisk the Dijon mustard and lemon juice together for light dressing. Combine in a separate bowl, broccoli, cherry tomatoes and baby spinach. Add in garlic, oregano, red pepper flakes and toss together. Drizzle with olive oil and top with mustard dressing.

Cauliflower Broccoli Salad

1 head cauliflower
1 bunch broccoli
1 small onion, chopped
1 package frozen peas (or pea pods)

2 cups mayo
1 cup sour cream
1 tsp minced garlic

Directions:
Mix mayo, sour cream and minced garlic in a small bowl. Chop cauliflower and broccoli into bite sized florets. Add in chopped onion. Mix vegetables with sauce. Add peas last.

Cranberry Salad

1 can crushed unsweetened pineapple
1 tablespoon lemon juice
1 cup fresh cranberries – chopped fine
1 small orange – peeled and quartered
1 cup celery – chopped
2 cups of romaine lettuce, chopped
½ cup pecans or almonds, optional

Directions:
Drain pineapple, mix ½ cup pineapple juice with lemon juice to dress salad. Combine cranberries, oranges, and celery with romaine lettuce. Drizzle pineapple lemon dressing over salad and top with pecans or almonds.

Spicy Broccoli Pasta

12 ounces bow-tie pasta

2 tablespoons extra virgin olive oil

2 garlic cloves, thinly diced

2 cups distilled water

1/4 teaspoon of red-pepper flakes

1 head broccoli florets, sliced

1/2 cup Parmesan cheese, grated

Directions:
Bring distilled water to a boil and cook bow-tie pasta until al dente. Drain and return to pot.

In a large pan, heat olive oil over a medium heat. Slowly add diced garlic and red-pepper flakes and stir until garlic is a golden color and soft. Add broccoli and 1/2 cup distilled water and season with salt and pepper. Cover pot; allow broccoli to soften, about 10 minutes. Add pasta to broccoli mixture, sprinkle with Parmesan.

Asian Style Pasta

3 tablespoons soy sauce

3 tablespoons rice vinegar

2 tablespoons smooth peanut butter

1 tablespoon honey

3 cloves garlic, minced

2 tablespoons minced fresh ginger

2 eggplants, 1 pound each, peeled and cut into 1/2-inch chunks

8 ounces snow peas, strings removed, halved diagonally

2 red bell peppers, ribs and seeds removed, cut into 1/2-inch-wide strips

8 ounces Pappardelle-type pasta noodles

Directions:

In large bowl, combine soy sauce, vinegar, garlic, and ginger; next, add in peanut butter and honey, then set aside.

Steam eggplant in a basket, over a pan of simmering water; cover, and allow eggplant to become tender, turning occasionally, about 15 minutes. Add the snow peas and red bell peppers; cook until tender but still crisp. Remove basket with eggplant from pan.

In a pot of boiling water, cook pasta until al dente. Drain and add pasta to steamed vegetables and toss with dressing mixture. Toss evenly.

Cannery Row Soup

Choose 2 lb. fish fillets (such as flounder, sole, haddock); slice into chunk cubes

2 tablespoons extra virgin olive oil

1 clove garlic, minced

3 carrots cut in thin strips

1 cup of celery, chopped

1/2 cup yellow onions, chopped

1/4 cup green peppers, chopped

1 (28 oz.) can whole tomatoes, cut up

1 cup clam juice

1/4 tsp. dried thyme leaves

1/4 tsp. dried basil, crushed

1/8 tsp. black pepper

1/4 cup fresh parsley, minced

Directions:

Heat olive oil in large saucepan over medium heat. Sauté the minced garlic, onion, sliced celery, chopped green pepper, and carrot strips in olive oil for about 3 minutes. Add remaining ingredients, except for the fish fillets and the parsley. Cover, lower heat and allow to simmer until vegetables are fork tender, about 15 minutes. Add fish and parsley. Cover and simmer for 5–10 minutes more or until fish flakes easily and is opaque.

Comforting Minestrone Soup

1/4 cup extra virgin olive oil

1 clove garlic, minced

1 1/3 cup onion, chopped

1 1/2 cup celery, coarsely chopped

1 can (6 oz.) tomato paste

1 tablespoon fresh parsley, chopped

1 cup carrots, sliced, fresh or frozen

3 cups cabbage, shredded

1 can (1 lb.) tomatoes, cut up

1 cup canned red kidney beans, rinsed and drained

1 ½ cup frozen peas

1 ½ cup of fresh green beans

10 cups distilled water

2 cups macaroni elbows, uncooked

Directions:

Heat olive oil in small saucepan. Add garlic, onion, and celery and sauté until tender, for about 5 minutes. Add all remaining ingredients except elbow macaroni. Stir until ingredients are blended. Bring to boil then reduce heat, cover, and simmer for about 45 minutes. Add uncooked macaroni and simmer for only 2–3 minutes.

Spicy Bar-b-cue Chicken

5 Tablespoon tomato paste
1 teaspoon ketchup
2 teaspoon raw honey
1 teaspoon molasses
1 teaspoon Worcestershire sauce
4 teaspoon white vinegar
3/4 teaspoon cayenne pepper

1/8 tsp black pepper
1/4 tsp onion powder
2 cloves garlic, minced
1/8 tsp ginger, grated
1 1/2 lb chicken (breasts, drumsticks), skinless

Directions:

Combine all ingredients in a medium sized pan and simmer for 15 minutes. Clean chicken and lightly pat dry. Place chicken in deep dish and rub with half of sauce mixture. Cover with saran wrap and marinate in refrigerator for 2 hours. Turn oven to 350 ° F. Pour remaining sauce over chicken, then cover with aluminum foil and bake for 30 minutes.

Chicken Ratatouille

1 tablespoon extra virgin olive oil
4 medium-sized chicken breast, boneless, skinned, cut into 1-inch pieces
2 unpeeled zucchini, sliced thin
1 purple eggplant, peeled
1 medium onion, thinly sliced
1 can (16 oz) whole stewed tomatoes

1 medium green pepper, cut into 1-inch pieces
1/2 lb fresh shitake mushrooms, sliced
1 clove minced garlic
1 1/2 teaspoon crushed basil, dried
1 tablespoon fresh parsley, minced

Directions:

Heat olive oil in large nonstick skillet. Add chicken breasts and sauté on each side for about 10 minutes. Add zucchini, eggplant, onion, green pepper, and shitake mushrooms and cook until vegetables are tender - about 15 to 20 minutes; stir occasionally. Add tomatoes, minced garlic, basil, parsley, and pepper. Continue to cook until chicken is tender and thoroughly done – about 5 to 10 more minutes.

Turkey Stuffed Cabbage

1 whole head Green or Savoy cabbage
½ lb leanest ground beef
½ lb ground turkey
1 small yellow onion, minced
1 small yellow onion, sliced
1 can (16 oz) diced tomatoes

1 slice whole grain bread, torn apart
¼ cup distilled water
1/8 teaspoon ground black pepper
1 medium carrot, peeled and sliced
1 tablespoon lemon juice
2 tablespoon SPLENDA brown sugar
1 tablespoon cornstarch

Directions:
Rinse and chop cabbage. Carefully peel ten of its outer leaves and situate in saucepan. Cover with boiling distilled water and simmer for 5 minutes. Remove the cooked cabbage leaves and drain on paper towel. Take ½ cup of cabbage, shred and set aside. Brown the lean ground beef, ground turkey, and onion. Drain fat. Mix together all meat mixtures, bread crumbs, distilled water, and black pepper. Drain can of tomatoes and add to meat mixture. Mix well; place about 1/4 cup of the mixture on each cabbage leaf, then fold and place in skillet. Cover and allow to simmer slowly for about 1 hour until cabbage is tender. Mix lemon juice, cornstarch and brown sugar in small bowl and pour over stuffed cabbage rolls.

Easy Zucchini Parmesan

2 cups thinly sliced zucchini
1 tablespoon. water
1 teaspoon salt
3 tablespoon. grated parmesan cheese

1 small onion, chopped
2 tablespoons, extra virgin olive oil
Freshly ground pepper

Directions:

Place olive oil in pan over medium heat. Place all ingredients, except parmesan cheese in pan, cover and cook for about 2 minutes. Turn heat down to low, uncover and continue cooking and turning with wide spatula until al dente, about 5 minutes. Sprinkle with cheese and black pepper.

Penne Pasta Classic

1 lb. penne pasta
8 plum tomatoes
1/2 cup olives (black), pitted and sliced
1 bunch fresh basil

3 cloves fresh garlic, peeled
1 tablespoon extra virgin olive oil
1 tablespoon balsamic vinegar

Directions:

Wash and dry basil leaves and place in a blender with garlic, olive oil and vinegar. Blend until smooth. Cook penne in boiling water, drain and rinse in cold water. Add penne pasta to basil leaves mixture. Stir and keep warm on stove. Slice plum tomatoes lengthwise in 1/8 inch pieces.

In separate skillet, lightly sauté the tomatoes and olives over medium heat for 3 minutes and add this to pasta. Serve with grated cheese.

Broccoli Soup

1½ pounds broccoli, cut into small florets
1 large yellow onion, coarsely chopped
2 medium potatoes, sliced
2 cups vegetable or chicken stock

¼ teaspoon freshly squeezed lemon juice
¼ cup basil, chopped
Pepper to taste
1 cup cream, raw

Directions:

In a large pot, set heat to medium and combine the broccoli, chopped onion, sliced potatoes, vegetable stock, lemon juice, salt, and pepper and allow to boil. Turn the heat down to low, cover and simmer. Cook for about 25 minutes until the vegetables become tender. When soup is complete, add cream and blend ingredients. Sprinkle the rest of basil on top.

Spicy Miso Soup

1 medium coarsely chopped onion
3 cloves minced garlic
1 tablespoon coconut oil
1 teaspoon curcumin
½ teaspoon cayenne pepper
2 quarts vegetable stock
1 teaspoon garam masala

1 cup distilled water
1 bunch kale, chopped
2 cans garbanzo beans
1 can coconut milk
2 tablespoons white miso paste
¼ cup chopped cilantro

Heat coconut oil over medium heat and sauté onions and garlic until tender. Add in the curcumin, cayenne pepper, and masala. Let mixture cook for 3 minutes. Add the vegetable stock and cilantro and allow to simmer for about 5 minutes.

Add the kale, a little at a time until it will fit, then simmer for 5 minutes. Take a perforated spoon and proceed to take out most of the kale from pot and place in a blender; add ¾ of the garbanzo beans and 1 cup of distilled water. Blend lightly then return to the pan.

Add all the beans together with the coconut milk and simmer. Ladle a small amount of soup and place in a small bowl. Dissolve the miso paste in that soup and then transfer back into the soup pot.

Wild Rice Gourmet Salad

¾ cup wild rice
¼ cup brown rice
1 cup toasted walnuts, chopped
4 tablespoons extra virgin olive oil
2 tablespoons balsamic vinegar

1 teaspoon Dijon mustard
1 clove garlic, minced
¾ cup dried cranberries
½ cup chopped parsley
⅓ cup chopped scallions

Directions:

In a medium-sized saucepan bring 2 cups of water to a boil. Stir in both the wild and brown rice, allow to boil then reduce the heat to low. Cover the saucepan and cook on low for 45 minutes, or until all the water is absorbed.

Preheat oven to 400°F. Spread a single layer of walnuts on a baking sheet and toast until lightly browned, about 5 minutes. In a separate bowl, stir together extra virgin olive oil, vinegar, mustard and garlic. Remove rice from heat and place into a large bowl. Add the toasted nuts and cranberries to the rice; Toss everything with oil mixture and stir to cover completely. Top with parsley and scallions and cover, then refrigerate until chilled.

Sausage Stuffed Mushrooms

1 lb. mushrooms
½ lb. ground pork sausage
¼ cup onion, chopped
1/3 cup catsup

2 tablespoons soft bread crumbs
1 tablespoon dried parsley
1 tablespoon minced garlic
½ tablespoon dried basil

Directions:

Remove stems from mushrooms and chop; you'll need 1/2 cup. In a skillet over medium-high heat, brown the sausage, mushroom stems and chopped onion, stirring frequently to avoid sticking. Drain grease off meat mixture and place in a bowl; add in catsup, bread crumbs, garlic, basil and parsley. Spoon the mixture into each mushroom cap. Assemble mushroom caps on a baking sheet and place in oven uncovered, at 350 degrees for about 12 to 15 minutes.

White Chicken Chili

2 onions, chopped
1 tablespoon virgin olive oil
6 cups chicken broth
3 16oz cans Great Northern beans, drained and rinsed
3 5-oz. cans chicken, drained
2 4-oz. cans diced green chiles

2 teaspoon ground cumin
1 tablespoon minced garlic
1-1/2 tablespoon dried oregano
1/4 teaspoon white pepper
12-oz. container sour cream
3 cups shredded Monterey Jack cheese

Directions:
Sauté onions in olive oil, over medium heat, until tender. Stir in your remaining ingredients except for the Monterey Jack cheese and sour cream. Reduce heat; simmer for 30 minutes, stirring frequently, until heated through. Shortly before serving time, top with sour cream and Monterey jack cheese. Stir until cheese is melted.

Roasted Veggie Salsa

4 Roma tomatoes
1 large zucchini
1 large yellow squash
1 large red bell pepper
1/4 large eggplant (optional)
1 cup corn kernels (fresh or frozen)
1/4 cup red onion, finely diced
1/2 tablespoon turmeric
1/2 tablespoon ground cumin
1/8 teaspoon liquid smoke (optional, but fantastic)
1/4 cup orange juice
Salt and pepper, to taste

Directions:

Preheat your oven to 450°F. Halve the tomatoes lengthwise, and quarter the zucchini, squash and bell pepper lengthwise. Roast until softened then add the corn after about 15 minutes. Remove from oven, and let cool. Next, dice vegetables and place in a large bowl. Mix in diced onion, spices, and orange juice. Adjust seasonings and salt and pepper to taste. Cover and allow to chill for at least 30 minutes.

Eat with crackers or as the filling in a sandwich wrap.

Split Pea Soup

2 cups diced yellow onions
4 cloves garlic, minced
1 16-ounce bag split peas, picked and rinsed
2 bunches of fresh carrots, peel and chop into fourths
3 cups white potatoes, peel and dice
6 cups vegetable broth
Ground black pepper
1/4 teaspoon salt
1 cup distilled water

Directions:

In a large pot, place diced onions and minced garlic with a small bit of water and allow to simmer until tender. Place all other ingredients into the pot, cover and allow ingredients to come to a boil. Turn heat down and allow to simmer. Cook for 45 minutes, stirring occasionally.

Tomato Soup

1 quart whole, canned tomatoes
¼ cup diced onion
2 sprays parsley
½ bay leaf.

½ teaspoon black pepper
3 tablespoons unsalted butter
2 tablespoons soy flour

Directions:

Cook the tomatoes, diced onion, parsley and bay leaf together for 20 minutes, then strain. Melt butter in a sauce pan, add soy flour and stir to a smooth paste, allow soup to cook for one minute; thin the soup out a bit with tomato mixture until it has a consistency that pours. Combine the ingredients (both mixtures).

Baked Dijon Salmon

1/4 cup unsalted butter, melted
1 1/2 tablespoons raw honey
1/4 cup dry whole grain bread crumbs
4 teaspoons chopped fresh parsley

3 tablespoons Dijon mustard
1 tablespoon minced garlic
4 (4 ounce) fillets salmon
1 juiced lemon

Directions:

Preheat oven to 400 degrees F. Stir together butter, mustard, and honey in a small bowl and set aside. In a separate bowl, mix the bread crumbs and parsley. Brush each salmon fillet with the Dijon mustard and honey mixture, and then sprinkle the bread crumb mixture on top.

Bake the Dijon salmon about 15 minutes. Squeeze the lemon gently over top of fillets and season with salt and pepper.

Marrakesh Vegetable Curry

1 sweet potato, peeled and cubed
1 medium purple eggplant, cubed
2 carrots, chopped
1 yellow onion, finely chopped
6 tablespoons extra virgin olive oil
3 cloves minced garlic
1 teaspoon ground curcumin
1 tablespoon curry powder
1 teaspoon cinnamon
½ tablespoon sea salt
½ teaspoon cayenne pepper
1 (15 ounce) can garbanzo beans, drained
1/4 cup almonds, lightly blanched
1 zucchini, sliced
2 tablespoons golden raisins
1 cup non-pulp orange juice
10 ounces spinach

Directions:

In a large heavy bottomed pot place eggplant, red and green peppers, carrots, sweet potato, yellow onion, and three tablespoons olive oil; sauté over a medium heat for 5 minutes. Heat a medium-sized pan with 3 tablespoons extra virgin olive oil, minced garlic, curry powder, cinnamon, curcumin, salt and pepper and sauté for 3 minutes. Next, place the garlic and spice mixture into the pot with vegetables in it. Add the beans, blanched almonds, zucchini, golden raisins, and non-pulp orange juice. Simmer slowly, for about 20 minutes while covered. Next, begin to place spinach into the pot and cook for about 5 more minutes.

Quick and Light Asparagus Soup

1 can of asparagus, rinsed and drained
1 can of condensed cream of chicken soup
½ teaspoon minced fresh ginger

½ teaspoon minced garlic
1 cup distilled water
Toasted whole wheat bread

Directions:

In a small saucepan, combine asparagus, cream of chicken soup, 1 cup distilled water, garlic and ginger. Bring to simmer and cook for 10 minutes. Transfer to blender and puree lightly. Serve with whole wheat toast.

Thai Butternut Soup

2 pounds butternut squash, peeled and diced
2 tablespoons red curry paste
1 ¼ cups coconut cream
¼ cup chopped cilantro
Salt and pepper to taste

Directions:
Sauté squash and red curry paste in medium pan. Add coconut cream to deglazed pan, top with enough water to be level with squash and bring to boil. Reduce heat, simmer until squash becomes soft. Place in blender and puree lightly, then season with salt and pepper and top with cilantro.

Loaded Baked Potato

2 baking potatoes
¼ cup cottage cheese
1 tablespoon minced garlic

1 tablespoon green onion
Shredded cheddar cheese

Directions:
Preheat oven to 350F. Pierce potato with knife several times, then wrap in foil. Bake for 40 minutes, or until soft. Remove; let stand for 5 minutes. Remove foil, cut a crisscross into the potato and sprinkle all ingredients on top. Top off with cheddar cheese and lastly, cottage cheese.

Mediterranean Chickpea Salad

1 cup of dried chickpeas, soaked overnight
½ cup sesame paste
1 tablespoon dark sesame oil

½ teaspoon ground cumin
Juice of 2 lemons
¼ garlic clove, minced

Directions:
Add chickpeas to saucepan with water to cover. Bring to boil, cover and simmer until chickpeas are very tender, about 30 minutes. Remove from heat and drain, reserve ¼ cup of liquid. Transfer chickpeas and the reserved liquid to a blender and mix with brief bursts until chickpeas are coarse and grainy.
Combine the puree in a bowl with the sesame paste, cumin and lemon juice and stir. Add in garlic. Drizzle with sesame oil. Can also be served on toasted crackers.

Mango Salsa Patties

Grated zest and juice of ½ lime
½ jalapeno pepper, seeded and chopped
1 cup mango, peeled and cubed
3 sprigs cilantro, finely chopped

1 cup crushed whole wheat crackers
1 pound lean ground beef
3 tablespoons extra virgin olive oil

Directions:
To make salsa, combine lime, jalapeno pepper, mango cubes and cilantro and mix well. Set aside.
Next combine beef, mango salsa and crushed cracker crumbs. Shape into medium patties. Heat a large skillet over medium heat and add olive oil. Add the patties and cook about 5 minutes on each side. Drain on paper towels.

Dinner Recipes

Stuffed Chicken Breasts

2 whole chicken breasts, skinned
1 cup carrots, shredded and chopped
1 cup zucchini, shredded
1 teaspoon sea salt

½ teaspoon poultry seasoning
1 packet of chicken bouillon
¼ cup distilled water

Rinse chicken and remove skin and excess fat from breasts. Slit the side of each breast along breastbone and remove breastbone. Take the tip of a sharp knife and cut the side of each chicken breast half, then cut and scrape the meat away from the rib cage; proceed to gently pull back meat to form a pocket, and then set aside.

Combine the chopped carrots, shredded zucchini, sea salt and poultry seasoning in a medium-sized bowl. Next, spoon mixture into each pocket of chicken – about 1/2 cup – then secure with toothpicks to hold. In a medium-sized skillet, place each stuffed chicken and sprinkle with chicken bouillon. Add the ¼ cup of distilled water over medium-to-high heat, and allow to boil. Turn heat down to low setting; simmer, covered for about 40 minutes or until chicken is tender. Remove toothpicks before serving.

Butternut Squash Curry

1 cup long grain brown rice
5 cups distilled water
2 small butternut squash, peeled and halved
1 large onion, cubed
4 garlic cloves
2 tablespoons tomato paste

¼ teaspoon crushed red pepper flakes
1 tablespoon safflower oil
1 tablespoon mustard seeds
¼ teaspoon ground coriander
1 teaspoon fennel seeds
1 teaspoon ground ginger

Directions:
Place rice in a medium saucepan with 2 cups distilled water and bring to boil; stir to avoid sticking, and reduce heat. Simmer uncovered until rice is tender and water is absorbed.
Cut squash into sections of large chunks. Puree onion, garlic and 1 tablespoon distilled water in blender until smooth. Heat safflower oil in a heavy bottomed pot, over medium heat. Add mustard and fennel seeds then coriander; cook and continue to stir about 2 minutes. Stir in ginger and cook, stirring often for about 10 minutes. Add tomato paste and cook for 2 minutes while stirring. Stir in remaining water and red pepper flakes. Add in the squash and bring to a boil. Turn down heat and allow to simmer for about 15 minutes. Spoon curried squash mixture over rice.

Lamb Shanks with Mushrooms and Cauliflower

4 lamb shanks
1 cup red wine
2 cups stock (lamb or vegetable)
2 tablespoons tomato paste
½ teaspoon dried oregano
3 sprigs chopped thyme

½ teaspoon ground cumin
3 tablespoons apple cider vinegar
¼ teaspoon cayenne pepper
4 cloves minced garlic
4 tablespoons olive oil
8 medium shitake mushrooms, sliced

Directions:
Marinate lamb shanks in red wine overnight or for a minimum of 4 hours. When lamb is removed, reserve marinade. In a heavy bottomed pot, brown the lamb in the extra virgin olive oil. Drain off oil. Add stock, tomato paste, and reserved marinade. Bring to boil; begin to skim. Add in the rest of the seasonings, but keep salt and pepper for last.

Bake lamb shanks at 300°F degrees for about 3 ½ hours or until lamb shanks are tender off the bone. About an hour before the end of baking put cauliflower florets and mushrooms in pot situated around the lamb. Remove the meat and cauliflowers, and set aside. Bring sauce to a boil and allow sauce to reduce by about half; allow it to thicken. Cover meat and veggies with sauce.

Spaghetti Casserole

12-oz. package spaghetti
1 lb. lean ground beef
1 cup onion, chopped
1 chopped bell green pepper
1 (28-oz.) can tomatoes, diced
4-oz. mushrooms, sliced

3.8-oz. can sliced black olives, drained and rinsed
2 teaspoons dried oregano
2 cup cheddar cheese, divided and shredded
10-3/4 oz. can cream of mushroom soup
1/4 cup distilled water
1/4 cup Parmesan cheese, grated

Directions:
Boil spaghetti in lightly salted water, al dente, and then set aside. Over medium heat, take a large skillet and brown ground beef, chopped onion and green bell pepper; drain oil off. Add shitake mushrooms, sliced black olives, tomatoes and oregano to skillet. Reduce heat to low and simmer, uncovered, for about 10 minutes. In a lightly greased baking pan, place half of the spaghetti. Place half of ground beef mixture on top of spaghetti. Sprinkle with one cup of Cheddar cheese. Repeat layers. Mix can of mushroom soup and distilled water until smooth; pour over top. Top with the grated parmesan cheese and bake at 350 degrees for 30 to 35 minutes, uncovered.

Stewed Beef Dumplings

1/4 cup soy flour
1 tsp salt
1/8 teaspoon pepper
2 lbs stewing beef cubed (or round steak, or blade steak)
6 slices of turkey bacon, broken up
3 medium onions, chopped
3 tsp salt
1/4 tsp pepper
1/8 tsp marjoram
2 clove garlic crushed
1/2 whole celery, chopped
6 carrots cut in bite-sized pieces
1 small turnip

Dumplings
2 cups soy flour
4 tsp baking powder
1/2 tsp salt
2 tablespoon margarine
1 cup distilled water or milk

Directions:
Combine soy flour, salt, and pepper in a dish, and then roll cubes of meat in mixture. Place turkey bacon pieces in a frying pan or saucepan and cook over a medium heat until transparent Add onions and celery. Add meat and brown lightly on all sides stirring constantly. Add the pepper, garlic, water, marjoram and bring to a boil, turn down heat, cover tightly and simmer till meat is nearly tender (1 1/2 to 2 hours)
Dumplings: mix all the dry ingredients together; add the margarine and water. If stew is to the top of pot pour off some liquid to start dumplings on top. Place small spoonfuls of dough on the top of stew and allow space for the dumplings to rise.

Baked Pineapple Rice Casserole

1 14oz can Pineapple chunks
1 tablespoon unsalted butter
2 ½ cups distilled water
¾ tablespoon salt

Directions:
Cook 1 cup of white rice in boiling water with 1 tablespoon of melted butter; turn down to low heat and cook with tight fitting lid for 20-30 minutes. Drain a can of pineapple chunks. Place 1/3 the rice in a buttered baking dish and cover with 1/2 the pineapple chunks. Repeat the layers then bake on 325F for about 20 minutes.

Easy Lentil Carrot Stew

1 (16-ounce) bag lentils
3 tablespoons ketchup
1 cup finely diced onions
3 cloves minced garlic
2 bay leaves

3 cups sliced carrots
4 cups vegetable broth
½ teaspoon dried thyme
1 15-ounce can of tomato sauce
2-1/4 cups distilled water

Directions:
Sauté onions and minced garlic in a little distilled water. Next, add the rest of the ingredients and bring mixture to a boil. Turn heat to low and allow pot to simmer for 1 hour or until lentils are soft.

Alphabet Soup

2 tablespoons olive oil
1 small sweet onion, chopped
2 carrots, sliced
1-2 cloves garlic, crushed
2 celery stalks, including leaves, sliced
2 tablespoons mixed Italian seasoning (buy packet)
1 15.5-ounce can kidney beans, rinsed well
1 28-ounce can crushed tomatoes
4 cups distilled water
1 cup alphabet-type pasta

Directions:
Heat olive oil on medium heat, in a large, soup pot. Add sweet onion, celery, carrots, crushed garlic and Italian seasonings. Sauté all vegetables until tender; about 10 to 15 minutes. Add crushed tomatoes, kidney beans, and distilled water, then bring to a boil. Add pasta and simmer soup until pasta is tender.

Sablefish with Bok Choy

2 tablespoons safflower oil
2 tablespoons ground ginger
3 garlic cloves, thinly sliced
1 head of bok choy, sliced crosswise
2 celery stalks, quartered

1 bunch scallions
2 tablespoons hoisin sauce
1 ½ Dijon mustard
1 teaspoon fresh lemon juice
4 Sablefish fillets

Directions:
In a large saucepan, heat safflower oil over medium-low heat. Add garlic and sprinkle ginger, stirring for 1 minute. Add sliced bok choy and chopped celery. Cook, stirring frequently until bok choy is crisp yet tender. Add scallions and continue stirring until bok choy is wilted.

Stir hoisin, mustard and lemon juice together and brush both sides of sablefish with mixture. Heat broiler on 350F and broil fish until cooked, about 7 minutes. Serve with side of bok choy.

Caponato

1 medium-large purple eggplant, cut into, 1-inch pieces

1/4 cup extra virgin olive oil

1 stalk of celery, chopped

1 bell pepper, red, chopped into ½ inch pieces

1 bell pepper, green, chopped into ½ inch pieces

1 medium-sized onion, coarsely chopped

3 tablespoons golden raisins

1/4 cup red wine vinegar

2 tablespoon capers, drained

2 garlic cloves, minced

1 (14oz) can diced tomatoes

2 teaspoons SPLENDA sugar substitute

1/2 teaspoon dried oregano leaves

Salt and pepper

Directions:

Slice up the eggplant and spread in a single layer, over a few layers of paper towels. Sprinkle with salt to cover each eggplant and toss around to coat all sides; spread evenly in one layer, then cover with another layer or two of towels. Heat the olive oil in a heavy large pan, over medium heat. Add the celery to the hot oil and sauté tender. Add half the onion and the eggplant and fry about 2 more minutes. Season with salt and pepper; add the bell peppers and cook about 3 more minutes. Add the remaining onion and cook until translucent, about 3 minutes. Over a medium heat, add the can of diced tomatoes, golden raisins, and oregano and let simmer until well blended and thickened. Stir often for about 20 minutes. Mix vinegar, SPLENDA, and capers and pour over caponato.

Easy Potato-Cheese Casserole

2 lb. package frozen hash brown potatoes (partially thawed)

2 cups shredded cheddar cheese

1 cup soy milk

1 small onion, minced

Salt and pepper to taste

Directions:
Combine hash brown potatoes, soy milk, and 1 small chopped onion; pour into greased baking dish and add salt and pepper. Top with minced onion. Cover and cook 300F for 1 hour.

Irish Corn Beef & Cabbage

4 pounds corned beef brisket
3 large cloves garlic, minced
1 tsp whole black peppercorns
12 small red potatoes small wedges

1 large onion, cut into wedges
Distilled water
1 beer

Directions:
Place corned beef in large pot and add 1 bottle of beer. Add distilled water and cover the corned beef. Add the spices (many times a spice packet will accompany the corned beef). Place minced garlic and black peppercorns in. Cover the pot and bring to a boil. Once at a boil, reduce to a simmer. Simmer approximately 4 hours (about 1 hour per pound) or until tender. Add the potatoes, carrots and turnips 1 hour before your corned beef is finished cooking (after about 3 hours of simmering). Add cabbage and onion then continue to cook for just 15 more minutes. Remove from heat and let everything rest for 15 minutes.

Slow Cook Beef & Cabbage

2 lb. lean ground beef
1 small head cabbage, shredded
1 small onion, chopped
1 (16 oz.) can stewed tomatoes
2 garlic cloves, crushed

1 teaspoon sea salt
1 teaspoon thyme
1 red bell pepper, diced
1 green bell pepper, diced
1 tablespoon oregano

Directions:
Brown ground beef and onions in a medium pan, and drain off fat. Pour the can of tomatoes into bottom of crock pot and begin layering the ingredients; cabbage, then spices, then meat and onion mixture, and garlic cloves. Create layers of both meat and then cabbage. When finished with layers, place last of stewed tomatoes on top. Cook on medium heat for 2 hours. Stir well to blend and then simmer on low and cook for 4 hours.

Greek Stew

3 cups lean stew beef
3 small yellow onions
3 cloves garlic, minced
1 (28 oz) can tomatoes
½ cup beef stock
1 small can tomato paste
2 tablespoon red wine vinegar

2 teaspoon dried oregano
½ teaspoon salt
½ teaspoon black pepper
½ cup soy flour
½ cup cold distilled water
1 sweet green pepper, chopped
½ cup crumbled feta cheese

Directions:
Place stew beef and chopped onions into soup pot and add garlic and tomatoes. Combine beef stock, red wine vinegar, oregano, salt, and pepper and place in pot. Stir to blend. Cook on low heat for about 4 hours. Stir the soy flour and distilled water in a cup and then add mixture to pot; stir well to blend. Next, stir in your chopped green pepper. Cook on high until stew begins to thicken – about 15 to 20 minutes. Sprinkle with feta cheese.

Garlic Mashed Potatoes

2 lb. potatoes, (peeled and diced)
2 garlic Cloves, peeled and mashed
½ to ¾ cups heavy Cream

Unsalted Butter
Salt
Pepper to taste

Directions:

Boil the potatoes until they are fork-tender. Heat the butter and cream separately until they melt (remove from heat as soon as the cream starts boiling). Make a mixture of butter, cream potatoes, and garlic. Season the mixture with salt and pepper and mash it until the mixture turns fluffy.

Spicy Vegetable Rice

3 cups rice

1 potato

1 small cabbage

1 frozen package mixed vegetables

2 medium Onions (sliced)

½ cups green chili

1 tablespoon cashew nuts

1 cup fresh coriander (chopped)

5 ground cloves

2-3 tablespoons cinnamon

4-5 bay leaves

5-6 green cardamoms

2 tablespoons saffron seasoning

2 cloves   garlic minced

2 tablespoons garlic paste

1 teaspoon red chili powder

1 teaspoon tomato ketchup

1 cup coconut milk

1 cup thick curd

4 tablespoons cooking oil

Directions:

Wash the rice until water runs clear. Once done soak the washed rice in cold water for 30-45 minutes. Grind green chili, fresh mint and coriander leaves. Boil the vegetables such that they are not too soft. Heat the oil in an appropriate sized pot and add all the spices. Mix well then put in the sliced onions and fry the onions until they are golden brown. Once done, add the ginger and garlic paste and cook well.

Add the semi- boiled vegetables followed by the paste. Add coconut milk and water (coconut milk and water solution should be 4 cups for 3 cups of water). Add tomato ketchup, thick curd, red chili powder and salt mix well.

As soon as the mixture starts boiling add in the soaked rice. Cook on high heat with gentle stirring till the water is almost absorbed by the rice. At this point lower the heat to the minimum, cover the pot with a lid and cook for 10-15 minutes. Sprinkle saffron seasoning on top.

Indian Butter Chicken

1/4 pint natural yogurt

1 ½ teaspoon chili powder

1/4 teaspoon allspice

1/4 teaspoon ground cinnamon

1 teaspoon curry powder

1/4 teaspoon dried bay leaves

4 green cardamom shells

1 teaspoon ground ginger

2 teaspoon minced garlic

1 can stewed tomatoes

1 1/4 teaspoon salt

6 boneless, skinless chicken, cubed

3 tablespoons margarine

1 tablespoon safflower oil

2 onions sliced

2 tablespoon fresh chopped coriander

4 tablespoon fresh cream

Directions:

Blend together the yogurt and all the dry spices, ginger, garlic, tomatoes and salt in a bowl and mix thoroughly. Next, combine chicken and yogurt mixture in a bowl to marinate. Melt together the margarine and safflower oil in a medium frying pan and stir in sliced onions. Fry onions until tender for about 5 minutes, stirring so not to stick. Stir in the chicken and yogurt. Next, add in 1 tablespoon of the coriander and mix well. Combine all the mixtures and blend together. Sprinkle dish with the chopped coriander.

Fajita Pizza

2 Chicken Breast Halves (boneless & skinless cut into thin strips)

1 cup Colby Cheese (shredded)

1 cup Monterey Jack Cheese (shredded)

1 medium Capsicum (sliced into ½" strips)

1 medium Onion (cut into wedges)

1 clove Garlic (minced)

2 tablespoons Coriander Leaves

1 medium Red Bell Pepper (sliced into ½" strips)

¼ cup Salsa (for garnish)

2 teaspoon Fajita Seasoning

Sour Cream

½ cup Olive Oil

Whole-grain, store bought Pizza Dough

Directions:

Pre-heat oven to 450 degrees. Trim a baking paper so that it would fit your pizza pan. Place the pizza crust in the pan and mist the crust and the rim of the pan with olive oil. Cut the chicken, peppers and onions (preferable size ½ inch strips). Heat the chicken in olive oil till it's no longer pink. Once done, add the onions, garlic, fajita seasoning and bell peppers. Continue cooking till chicken is thoroughly cooked but the vegetables are tender crisp.

Remove from the heat and drain any water/juices and add the salsa. Sprinkle the Colby cheese on the pizza crust and arrange the mixture and sprinkle the Monterey jack cheese on top. Let the pizza bake for 12-14 minutes.

Grilled Trout

4 Brook Trout

2 tablespoon Parsley (chopped)

2 tablespoon Sesame Seeds

½ tablespoon Ginger

½ tablespoon Salt

¼ cup Lemon Juice

1 tablespoon Hot Sauce

2 tablespoon unsalted butter (melted)

2 tablespoon canola oil

Directions:

Form a mixture of hot sauce, salt, oil, lemon juice, parsley, sesame seeds, ginger and margarine. Cut into the fish with a sharp knife or blade and soak it in the mixture. Cover the soaked fish and refrigerate for an hour or so. Begin grilling the fish. Rotate trout so each side is grilled for 3-5 minutes and keep brushing/spraying the fish with lemon juice mixture.

Rice Kabsa

3 cups Wild Rice

3 Chicken Bouillon (cubes)

1 Onion, finely chopped

5 teaspoons minced garlic

1/2 cup Pine Nuts

1/2 cup Coconut Oil

5 ½ cups distilled water

Directions:

Lightly cook garlic, pine nuts and onions in the butter. When the mixture turns brown add water and chicken bouillon. When the water starts boiling add the rice, lower the heat and leave the mixture on the lowered heat for 15-20 minutes. Once the rice is ready remove from heat. Cook chicken the way you like it (grilled, boiled, baked) and mix.

Quick Vegetarian Dinner Wrap

1 tablespoon cooking oil

2 organic eggs

2 tablespoons cheese (optional)

1 tablespoon onion (diced)

1 slice tomato (diced)

1/2 tablespoon green pepper (diced)

2 leaves of Romaine lettuce

1 tablespoon of store-bought salsa

1 whole grain wrap

Directions:

Heat cooking oil in the pan on medium heat while whisking eggs. When pan is sufficiently hot, add the eggs. Slice the cheese. Once eggs are partially scrambled, add the diced vegetables and cheese to the pan. Next, add the salsa; Wash and slice lettuce. Add mixture in middle of whole grain wrap and fold.

Stove-Top Stuffed Potatoes

6 medium white potatoes, peeled
2 bunches of cauliflower florets, chopped
1 tablespoon onion, chopped
1 pepper, chopped
1 teaspoon peas
2 green chilies, chopped

4 Roma tomatoes, cubed
2 garlic cloves, chopped
1 tablespoon coriander leaves chopped
1/4th cup unsalted butter
2/3rd cup distilled water
Salt and pepper to taste

Directions:
Slice a thick slice from the top of the potato to form a thick slice that will later become the cap, and scoop carefully the flesh from the inside of the potato. Boil the cauliflower, pepper, onion, peas, garlic, chilies and salt in the pan. Continue cooking the mixture until none of the water is left. Divide the mixture between the potatoes and cover with the potato caps, secured in place using toothpicks. Heat the butter in a saucepan to cook salted tomatoes over moderate heat for 3-4 minutes.

Assemble the stuffed potatoes and place over the tomato mixture. Place a lid on the pan and allow potatoes to steam for approximately 12 minutes until they are tender.

Chicken Curry in Tomato Puree

3 tablespoons butter or margarine
1 Onion sliced thinly
2 cloves garlic, thinly sliced

1 tablespoon curry powder
1 tablespoon tomato puree
2-2 1/2 pounds chicken pieces

Directions:
Melt the butter or margarine in a frying pan. Sauté sliced onions in butter. Add sliced garlic to onions and sauté until onions are tender. Add tomato puree and curry powder and sauté an additional 3 minutes.

Place the chicken pieces into the mixture, cover with a lid and allow to continue cooking 45-50 minutes until chicken is cooked. Remove lid and sprinkle with lemon juice. Tip: Be sure to continue to stir contents of pan while cooking to ensure nothing sticks. Add water as needed to avoid sticking.

Campfire Salmon Fillets

1 cup brown sugar
1 cup extra virgin olive oil
1/2 cup soy sauce
2 tablespoons and 2 teaspoons lemon pepper
1 tablespoon and 1 teaspoon dried thyme

1 tablespoon and 1 teaspoon dried basil
1 tablespoon and 1 teaspoon dried parsley
2 teaspoons garlic minced
16 (6 ounce) salmon fillets

Directions:
Combine the brown sugar, extra virgin olive oil, soy sauce, lemon pepper, thyme, basil, parsley, and minced garlic in a gallon size plastic bag. Shake vigorously to combine all ingredients well. Place the salmon fillets in the bag and place in an ice chest for at least 3 hours.
Preheat oven. Remove the bag from the ice chest. Carefully remove the fillets from the sauce and discard the marinade. Insert fillets into broiler. Cook on each side for 8 minutes.

Indian Chicken Do Pyaaza

1 medium sized chicken
1/2 -1 teaspoon salt
2 tablespoon lemon juice
3/4 cup butter

4 large onions, chopped
2 crushed garlic cloves
2 cups yogurt
1 1/4th cups water

Spices

1 teaspoon red chilly powder
1 teaspoon turmeric powder
1/2-teaspoon ground ginger
2-3 pieces cinnamon stick

12 black peppercorns
1 brown cardamom
6 cloves

Garnish

1 teaspoon curry powder
1 cup peeled and halved cherry tomatoes

1 medium chopped onion, fried

Directions:

Cut chicken into chunks – about 8 pieces. Rub lemon juice and salt mixture into the chicken pieces. Place in refrigerator for 1/2 hour. Place butter in deep pan and heat, adding the cloves, cardamom, peppercorns and cinnamon sticks. Stir well and add the chicken along with the onion, garlic and other spices. Continue cooking over gentle heat for 15 minutes, stirring to prevent sticking.

Pour in yogurt and cook for 5 minutes using low heat and continually stirring. Add water, place lid on pan and cook an additional 40-45 minutes until chicken is done. Place in oven proof serving dish, sprinkle with curry powder and arrange tomatoes and onion around dish. Place dish in 300 degree F oven for 10-15 minutes.

Indian Fish Fillets

4 fish fillets
1/2 cup canola oil
1 tablespoon carom seeds
1/3 cup of fresh cream
2 teaspoons cumin seeds powder
2 teaspoons curry powder
1 tablespoon garlic paste
1/2 cup of flour

1/4 cup of lemon juice, or to taste
5 tablespoons mint sauce
1/2 teaspoon white pepper
1 onion, sliced
1 cup of yogurt
pinch of salt
1 tablespoon of chili powder

Directions:
Start with cooking the fish fillets. Dredge the fillets in the flour that has some of the garlic and spices added to it. Add the canola oil to a heated frying pan. Make sure that the oil is hot enough to fry the fish properly. Cook for about three minutes per side, taking care not to burn them. Turn off the heat and remove the fish from the pan once they are golden brown on both sides. Keep the fillets warm by placing them in the oven at low heat.
Mix the yogurt and cream together in a clean mixing bowl. Add the rest of the garlic, together with the spices, mint sauce and lemon juice. To serve, top the fillets with some onions and spoon some of the sauce over them. This dish will go well with steamed rice.

Spicy Red Corn Chowder

1 cup mushrooms
10 oz. package frozen corn
1 chili pepper
3 onions
1 cup chopped tomato
1 finger ginger
2 green chilies

1 tablespoon coriander leaves
1/2 lemon
1 garlic clove
1 teaspoon red chili powder
salt to taste
1/2 cup unsalted butter

Directions:
Rinse corn, drain and cook in pot with a little water to steam, then set aside. Cut each mushroom into 5-6 pieces. Chop onions finely and slice ginger thinly. Cut green chilies lengthwise in half. Chop tomatoes and chili pepper into cubes.
Chop coriander finely. Mince garlic. Heat butter in shallow pan and sauté onion until it becomes lightly browned. Add minced garlic, tomatoes and red chili powder.
Once mixture is cooked, add mushrooms and corn, then add chili pepper and lemon, sauté for one minute and remove pan from flame. Garnish using green chilies and coriander.

Stuffed Baked Tomatoes

5-6 large tomatoes
1 cup cottage cheese
1 onion chopped
Coriander, finely chopped
2 chopped green chilies
1/2 teaspoon turmeric powder

Curry powder to taste
Red chili powder to taste
1 teaspoon grated cheese
1 tablespoon oil
Pinch of salt

Directions:
Wash and dry tomatoes. Remove top of tomato to form a cap. Gently remove seeds and pulp from center of tomato. Set aside the portion removed and chop the tops. Place oil in pan and heat. Add green chilies and chopped onions, cooking until soft. Add some of the pulp and tops to the pan, cooking for a minute, then add the dry ingredients and cook one more minute. Add cottage cheese. Mix and heat for another minute. Use mixture to fill tomatoes. Top each tomato with grated cheese and chopped coriander. Bake in a 300 degree oven for 20 minutes.

Vegetable Biryani

1 cup Rice
1 cup Mixed Vegetable (beans, cauliflower, carrots, potatoes)
150 grams Green Peas
2 to 3 thinly Sliced Onions
1 Sliced Green chili
Salt to taste
1/2 teaspoon Red Chili Powder
1 teaspoon caraway Seeds, Cinnamon

3 Cloves
1/2 teaspoon Black Pepper Powder
3 Tomatoes
1/2 cup Yogurt
2 tablespoons Vegetable cooking Oil
1/2 teaspoon Mustard Seeds
2 tablespoon Dry Fruits (raisins, cashew nuts)

Directions:
Put rice in a washed bowl and place it aside. Take rice with 2 to 2 1/2 cups water and add a little salt and dry fruits. Prepare it in a pan/cooker. Shred vegetables into little thin pieces and fry them in cooking oil. Place oil in pan, add mustard seeds, powder, caraway seeds, cinnamon cloves, green chilies, black pepper and continue to stir for 30 seconds. Add onions and sauté all of it for about 1 minute, waiting until they are golden-pink. Add red chili powder and salt and continue to stir. Now put in the chopped tomatoes and fry it all until everything is cooked well.
Next blend the yogurt and be sure to make it smooth. Simmer for 15 - 20 seconds. Put all the vegetables you have already fried into the pan. Lastly, add the cooked rice in the bowl, and mix it up and cook it for about 3 - 5 minutes.

Rava Dosa

2 cups semolina
1/2 cup rice flour
1/2 cup buttermilk
2 tablespoons of whole garlic cloves, crushed
1 inch ginger
4 green chilies

3 tablespoons curry powder
1 quarter cup shredded coconut
12 cashew nuts
2 tablespoon peppercorns
1 teaspoon cumin seeds
2 tablespoons olive oil

Directions:
Blend rice flour, semolina, and buttermilk to create a thin batter. Set the batter aside for at least six hours. Wash and finely chop the curry leaves, ginger, and green chilies. Chop the cashew nuts and coconut into very little pieces and then squash cumin seeds and peppercorns.
Heat up the clarified butter and roast the peppercorn and cumin seeds, then add it to the mixture. Add in the chopped green chili, coconut, and cashews into the batter. Mix well. Pour a little oil and grease a non-stick pan. Take a scoop of the mixture and pour it while twirling the pan to spread the batter. Sprinkle 1 tablespoon olive oil over the dosa. Cook till it is golden brown and crisp.

Salmon Lemon Bake

1/2 teaspoon pepper
4 (6-7 ounce) salmon
1 teaspoon lemon juice

3 tablespoon. of mustard (Dijon)
3 tablespoon raw honey

Directions:
Place the lemon juice, mustard and honey in a small mixing bowl and stir. Put the salmon in a medium-sized baking dish, situated in a single layer. Take the mixture from the bowl and spread it evenly over each salmon steak. Sprinkle salt and pepper to taste. Allow to bake for around 20 minutes. Bake in the oven at 325 degrees.

Mix up a side salad served with dressing and croutons and a thick slice of your favorite bread for a complete meal.

Mediterranean Pasta and Shrimp

2 teaspoon olive oil

2 cloves garlic, minced

1 lb. large shrimp (already deveined and peeled)

2 cups chopped tomato

1/3 cup chopped olives

¼ teaspoon pepper

4 cups cooked pasta (angel hair)

¼ cup feta or parmesan cheese

Directions:

Heat oil in non stick pan over medium heat. Add shrimp and garlic, stirring slowly about two minutes. Add tomato, stir in gently and simmer mixture for 4 minutes. When tomatoes are softened, add olives and black pepper and stir. Combine cooked pasta and shrimp mixture into large bowl and stir well. Top with cheese and serve hot.

Mushroom Garlic Pasta

1 lbs of spaghetti

3 tbs of olive oil

½ lbs of fresh mozzarella cheese

2 tbs of freshly grated parmesan cheese

2 tbs of fresh chopped parsley

2 tbs of dried chopped tomatoes

1 cup sliced shitake mushrooms

2 tablespoons of minced garlic cloves

Salt and pepper

Directions:

Boil spaghetti in boiling salted water. Mix olive oil with minced garlic, chopped parsley and dried tomatoes. Drain the spaghetti and immediately toss it with the olive oil mixture. Add chopped mushrooms. Place spaghetti into a baking dish. Slice mozzarella cheese into large circles and place them over the pasta. Sprinkle grated parmesan cheese and freshly ground pepper. Bake at 345 degrees F for 20 minutes. Garlic bread sticks are a great addition to this recipe.

Halibut with lemon egg sauce

1 large onion

1 carrot pared and sliced

1 lb halibut steak

3/4 cups water

salt and pepper

juice and peeled rind of 1/4 lemon

For sauce:

2 teaspoons cornstarch
lemon
beaten egg

Garnish:

1/2 sliced cucumber
sliced lemon
parsley

Directions:

Put onions and carrots in skillet, place halibut on top, add seasonings, lemon juice and rinds, along with water. Cover, bring to a boil and simmer for fifteen minutes or until opaque. Place fish onto serving platter, reserving juice. Blend the cornstarch with the strained lemon juice. Bring the fish liquid to a boil and add to cornstarch mixture. Cook for 1 minute, slightly cool, pour into a bowl over the beaten egg. Mix and pour over fish.

Quick Mediterranean Dinner Wraps

1 tablespoon 1/3-less fat cream cheese

1 (9-inch) spinach or tomato basil wrap

3/4 cup chopped fresh baby spinach

1/2 avocado sliced

1/3 cup crumbled feta cheese

1/4 cup chopped tomato

2 tablespoon of sliced black olives

1 to 1 1/2 tablespoon chopped fresh basil

1 tablespoon wine vinaigrette

Directions:

Spread cream cheese over one side on the wrap. Top with chopped spinach and all remaining ingredients. Roll up the wrap tightly and cut diagonally in half.

Spinach Bowl with Olives and Pine Nuts

1 10-ounce bag fresh spinach with stems removed

2 Tablespoons of sliced black olives

2 teaspoons extra-virgin olive oil

2 cloves garlic, minced

1 Tablespoons pine nuts

2 Tablespoons golden raisins

2 teaspoons balsamic vinegar

1/8 teaspoons salt

1 Tablespoons grated Parmesan cheese

Freshly ground pepper to taste

Directions:

Heat the olive oil in a large non-stick pan over medium-high heat. Next add the minced garlic, pine nuts, and raisins. Continue stirring about 1 minute. Add the spinach and cook, stirring unit just wilted. Remove from the heat. Stir in the vinegar and salt. Serve right away with freshly grated pepper and Parmesan.

Mushroom Ciabatta

2 large portabella mushrooms, sliced into circles
1 tomato, sliced into circles
2 large balls of mozzarella cheese, sliced into circles
1 chopped onion
2 tablespoon. of olive oil
6 slices of toasted ciabatta bread
Salt and pepper

Directions:

Heat the olive oil in a frying pan and sauté mushrooms with onions for 3 minutes on each side. Place one portabella piece on each of the ciabatta bread servings. Garnish it with onions. Top it with a slice of mozzarella and sliced tomato. Sprinkle with salt and pepper to taste.

Seafood with Pasta Casserole

1 lbs of ziti pasta

1 lbs cooked shrimp

1 lbs cooked crab meat

½ chopped portabella mushrooms

1 chopped onion

2 tablespoon of minced garlic

1 tablespoon of dry Italian seasoning

3 tablespoon of freshly grated romano and parmesan cheese

2 tablespoon of extra virgin olive oil

Salt and pepper

Fresh parsley to garnish

Directions:

Cook the ziti according to the instructions on the package. Heat the olive oil in a frying pan; add the shrimp, the crab meat, mushrooms and onion. Sauté the ingredients for 5 minutes. Drain the pasta and toss it with the above mixture. Add minced garlic, Italian seasoning, 1 tablespoon of grated cheese. Place pasta into baking dish and sprinkle the top with the remainder of the grated cheese. Bake at 325 degrees for 20 minutes. Garnish with parsley.

Greek Oven Bake

1 package angel hair pasta

2 8 ounce cans of tomato sauce

1 cup sour cream

1/4 cup of marinated quartered artichoke hearts

3/4 cup crumbled feta cheese

1 can condensed cream of mushroom soup

1/4 cup of Greek olives, pitted and sliced in half

2 tablespoons of red onions, chopped

1/4 cup sun-dried tomatoes, sliced thin

3/4 teaspoons of dried oregano

1/4 teaspoon of pepper

Directions:

Cook pasta according to package directions. Pour the tomato sauce in a large bowl, then combine the remaining ingredients with the sauce. Drain pasta, then toss with sauce mixture. Transfer to a 1-1/2-quart casserole baking dish and coat with cooking spray. Bake for 30 to 35 minutes uncovered, at 375° or until heated through.

Chicken Snow Peas with Pasta

3 cups medium sized rotini or penne pasta, uncooked

1 lb. boneless chicken breast, cut into bite-sized pieces

¼ cup chopped onion

2 minced garlic cloves

½ cup sliced black olives

5 medium sized seeded and chopped tomatoes

1 cup fresh snow peas cut in half

3 Tablespoon. olive oil

Grated Parmesan cheese

Directions:
Cook pasta according to package. While it is cooking, prepare the rest of the ingredients. Heat olive oil in large non-stick frying pan on medium heat. Add onion and garlic. Cook for one minute. Add chicken. Cook for 5 minutes or until done. Stir occasionally.
Add snow peas, tomatoes, olives then reduce heat. Simmer until heated through. Stir occasionally. When finished, mix gently with cooked, hot pasta. Serve in 4 pasta bowls. Top each with Parmesan cheese to taste.

Indian Butter Chicken

1/4 pint natural yogurt
50 grams ground almonds
1 teaspoon chili powder
1/8 teaspoon crushed bay leaves
1/8 teaspoon ground cloves
1/8 teaspoon ground cinnamon
1/2 teaspoon curry powder

2 green cardamom shells
1/2 teaspoon ginger pulp

1/2 teaspoon garlic pulp
200 gram can of tomatoes
1 teaspoon salt
1/2 kg boned, skinned, and cubed chicken
45 g clarified butter
1/2 tablespoon corn oil
1 1/2 sliced onions
2 tablespoons freshly chopped coriander
2 tablespoons fresh cream

Directions:
Add almonds, yogurt, dry spices, tomatoes, garlic, ginger, and salt in a mixing bowl and blend it together. Place the chicken in another bowl and put the yogurt on top and marinate. Set aside the marinated chicken. Next, melt in a frying saucepan the clarified butter. Add onions and fry for four minutes. Add the chicken mixture and stir for about 8 - 10 minutes. Next add 1/2 of the coriander and mix. While placing fresh cream into it, blend well. Heat it until it boils.

Mediterranean Roasted Fennel with, Feta, Prawns and olives on Pasta

1 Lg. Fennel Bulb

1 lb. shelled and deveined prawns

½ cup pitted kalamata olives

1 tablespoon pernod

Salt and pepper to taste

½ cup crumbled Feta

8 oz. fettuccini

½ cup olive oil

Heat oven to 400. Trim Fennel bulb and slice lengthwise into 16 pieces. Toss to coat with olive oil and place on baking tray. Roast for approximately 30 minutes. Heat 2 qts. water to boiling and cook pasta until al dente. Drain and set aside. Heat 3 tablespoons of olive oil to medium in non-stick skillet and heat olives until they are puffy. Add shrimp and Pernod, then cook until pink on each side. Toss with fennel, feta and pasta and serve.

Mediterranean Chicken Pasta

2 tablespoon olive oil

1 pound boneless, skinless chicken breasts, diced

6-ounce jar marinated artichoke hearts, quartered and drained

1/2 cup julienned sundried tomatoes

2 tablespoon minced garlic

1/2 cup chicken broth

1/2 cup kalamata olives, pitted and chopped

7 ounce jar roasted red peppers, sliced

1 pound cooked angel hair pasta

1/4 cup fresh chopped basil

6 ounces fresh crumbled feta cheese

Directions:

Heat the olive oil in a large skillet until hot. Sauté the chicken until it is cooked through and lightly brown on the outside. Add artichoke hearts, tomatoes, garlic, chicken broth, olives and peppers to the pan. Cook for 5 minutes, stirring occasionally. Add the fresh basil and cook for 2 minutes. Pour chicken mixture over cooked pasta, tossing to coat. Add salt and pepper to taste. Sprinkle with feta cheese crumbles and serve hot.

Honey Soy Broiled Salmon

2 tablespoons soy sauce (reduced-sodium)

1 tablespoon white rice vinegar

1 tablespoon raw honey

1 teaspoon ground ginger

4 salmon fillets

1 green scallion, minced

1 teaspoon sesame seeds, lightly toasted

Directions:

Blend together the soy sauce, honey, scallion, vinegar, and ginger in an appropriately sized bowl until the honey is dissolved. Put salmon in a re-sealable plastic container, add 3 tablespoons of the mixture and refrigerate; let marinate for up to 15 minutes. Reserve what is left of the sauce for later. Preheat broiler, then place aluminum foil into a small baking pan - coat dish with cooking spray. This allows for easy cleanup.

Discard the marinade and place salmon fillets into pan, with skinned-side down. Broil fillets until cooked thoroughly - about six to ten minutes. Drizzle fillets with leftover sauce and garnish with sesame seeds.

Orzo with Olives and Feta

4 ounces lean ground lamb
1 ½ teaspoons extra virgin olive oil
1 large finely chopped yellow onion
1/4 cup crumbled feta cheese
3 cloves garlic, minced
1 teaspoon ground cinnamon
½ teaspoon oregano

1 can whole tomatoes, (14-ounce) un-drained
2 tablespoons black olives, pitted and chopped
Pinch of Salt and black pepper each
1 box (12 ounces) orzo pasta

Directions:
Brown lamb in a skillet over medium heat for about three to five minutes. Drain oil off lamb, place in separate bowl and set aside. In a medium heavy bottomed pot, heat the olive oil. Add chopped onion and sauté, stirring, until softened, four to five minutes. Add cinnamon, garlic, oregano; cook, stirring gently, until fragrant, about one minute more. Add the un-drained whole tomatoes to the meat and cook, stirring, until the sauce is thickened, about ten minutes then remove and set aside. Next, stir in black olives and garnish with pepper and salt. Cook orzo pasta in a pot of boiling water. Garnish dish with crumbled feta cheese.

Greek Beef & Peas

3 cups penne pasta, uncooked
1 lb. beef strips, trim into bite-sized pieces
¼ cup chopped shallots
3 minced garlic cloves
½ cup sliced black olives

5 medium sized seeded and chopped tomatoes
1 cup green peas and bite sized carrots
3 tablespoon olive oil
Grated Parmesan cheese

Directions:
Boil pasta in salted boiling water. While it is cooking, prepare the rest of the ingredients. Heat olive oil in large skillet on medium heat. Add shallots and garlic cloves. Cook until tender for about 2 minutes. Add beef strips. Cook for 5 minutes or until al dente. Stir occasionally. Add green peas, carrots, tomatoes, and olives. Reduce heat. Simmer until heated through. Stir occasionally. When finished, mix gently with cooked, hot pasta. Top each with Parmesan cheese to taste.

Lean Pork Chops over Rice

8 pork chops, cut into 3/4 inch sections

2 tablespoon Coconut oil

1 cup of uncooked rice

1 14.5 ounce can of chicken broth

1/2 cup of water

1 chopped onion

1 tablespoon minced garlic

1 10 ounce package of frozen peas

1/2 tablespoon salt

1/2 tablespoon dried thyme

Directions:

Place a large skillet on medium heat, then brown the pork chops with the coconut oil. Remove the pork, drain off the oil and toss in the rest of the ingredients.

Add in the pork chops over the top of the ingredients and bring the pot to a boil. Once boiling, reduce the heat to low and cover for 20 to 25 minutes. Check the rice after 20 minutes then remove from heat once tender.

Crockpot Pork Roast Dinner

1 lb. red potatoes, slice into wedges

16 oz. pkg. baby carrots

1 chopped yellow onion

2 cloves garlic, minced

3 lb. boneless pork loin roast

4 tablespoons Dijon mustard

1 teaspoon tarragon leaves

1/2 teaspoon salt

1/4 teaspoon pepper

1 ½ cups beef broth

Directions:

In a 4-6 quart crockpot, place potatoes and baby carrots around the bottom edge of the pot. Place the garlic and onions on the bottom of the crockpot. In a small bowl, mix the Dijon mustard, tarragon, salt, and pepper together. Take the mixture and spread it over the pork roast. Take the pork roast and place it in the crockpot, and then pour the beef broth all over the roast and vegetables. Let the entree cook for 8-9 hours or until the pork has reached 150 F and the vegetables are tender. Serve vegetables and pork on a platter, or let them sit with the covered lid for 15 minutes to prepare gravy using the broth. Take the broth, 1 - 1/2 tablespoons of cornstarch and 3 tablespoons of water, heat in sauce pan until it thickens, and serve.

Chinese Barbecue Spareribs

1 cup soy sauce
1 teaspoon salt
1 teaspoon curry powder
4 pounds of spareribs

1 tablespoon sugar

3 tablespoons red wine

1/2 cup water
1 mashed clove of garlic

Directions:

Clean and slit your ribs. Put ribs in large bowl. Mix all of the dry ingredients and rub into ribs and allow to marinate for 30 minutes in fridge. Next, combine soy sauce, water and red wine. Remove ribs and pour these wet ingredients on top of the ribs. Keep the liquid and use it to baste the ribs while they are grilling.

A grill is not needed to bake your ribs. This same recipe can be used to bake ribs in a 350 degree oven for an hour and a half.

Chicken with Panang Curry

5 Tablespoon curry paste

Cooking oil (canola or olive oil)

4 cups of coconut milk

2/3 lbs chicken breast, cut into cubes

2 tablespoon palm sugar

6 torn kaffir lime leaves

2 sliced chile peppers

1/4 fresh basil

Directions:

Cook the curry paste and oil in a large skillet set over medium heat. Toss in the coconut milk and bring the skillet to a boil. Once boiling, add in the chicken and stir until the chicken is cooked through.

Add in the palm sugar and lime leaves for about five minutes and salt to taste. Once cooking time is complete, remove from heat and serve with the red chile peppers and basil as garnishes sprinkled over.

Tofu and Basil over Brown Rice

5 chopped green onions

6 minced garlic cloves

1 package of tofu, drained and marinated in soy sauce over night

1 cup of chopped fresh basil

1 tsp red chili pepper sauce

1 tsp soy sauce

Cooked brown rice

Directions:

Cook the garlic in a pot set over medium-high heat until tender. You may use water, vinegar or vegetable stock to cook the garlic in. Once tender, add in the marinated tofu you let sit in the soy sauce overnight. Make sure to watch the tofu as it does burn easily. The cook time should range anywhere from 5 to 10 minutes. Toss in the chili pepper sauce, soy sauce and basil, then allow it to cook completely through. Remove the tofu and serve it over the brown rice.

Alfredo Italian Sausage Casserole

12 oz Fettuccini Pasta
12 oz mild ground Italian Sausage
2 cup Italian flavored croutons or
corn bread stuffing mix
2 tablespoons Grated Parmesan Cheese
2 tablespoons chopped parsley
1 cup chopped onion
1 cup chopped celery
1 tablespoons extra virgin Olive Oil
1 jar (15 oz) Alfredo Sauce
2 cup spinach, chopped
salt and pepper

Directions:

Cook Fettuccini according to package directions, drain, and set aside. In skillet over medium heat, sauté onions, celery, and Italian sausage in the olive oil until sausage is fully cooked. Drain and set aside.

Lightly coat a 10' casserole dish with olive oil. Toss together fettuccini and sausage mixture, croutons, (or stuffing mix), toss in parsley and spinach. Mix lightly then pour into casserole dish. Add alfredo sauce, sprinkle with Parmesan cheese, salt and pepper to taste. Bake at 350 degree for 30 minutes.

Vegan Jambalaya Oyster

3 stalks of organic celery, with leaves
1 organic red bell pepper
1 organic red onion
1 cup organic wild rice
1 cup vegetable stock

¼ teaspoon cayenne pepper
1 cup diced vegan chicken
4 oz organic oyster mushrooms
2 tablespoons organic olive oil
Tabasco sauce to taste

Directions:

Dice and/or julienne the vegetables. Use vegetable broth to cook the rice. When the rice is done, heat up the oil in a wok. Next, stir in vegan chicken and add Cayenne Pepper to taste. When done move the chicken to the side of the wok. Put all the uncooked vegetables in the wok. Add more Tabasco sauce to taste and stir together vegetables and vegan chicken. When the vegetables are ready add the cooked rice to the wok. Stir until rice and Tabasco sauce are thoroughly blended. Remove from wok and enjoy.

Chicken Veggie Curry Casserole

1 frying chicken, cut up, and skinned

2 medium onions, chopped

2 tablespoons butter

2 teaspoons curry powder

½ teaspoon cumin seeds, ground

¼ teaspoon turmeric

1 garlic clove, minced

1 pinch cayenne powder

¼ teaspoon dried coriander

1 teaspoon salt (or to taste)

White pepper to taste

1 ½ tablespoons sour cream

3 potatoes, peeled and chopped

Directions:

Preheat oven to 350 degrees. Using a large saucepan, sauté the onions in butter over low heat until golden. Add the seasonings and continue cooking and stirring for 5-6 minutes, watching to ensure they don't burn. Add 1/8 cup of water and cook for another minute. Add the chicken pieces and sour cream. Cook for 10 -12 minutes to brown the chicken on all sides. Add another 1/8 cup of water. Add the potatoes and stir to coat with seasonings. Transfer all to a shallow casserole dish. Cover and bake in oven for 30 – 45 minutes, or until potatoes are cooked and chicken reaches an internal temperature of 165 degrees.

Tofu Ginger & Garlic

3 Tablespoons Canola Oil
2 Teaspoons Garlic Cloves, Minced
1 whole Lime

1 Tablespoon Soy Sauce, any brand
2 Teaspoons Minced Ginger Root
2 Pounds Firm Tofu, cubed

Directions:

Heat your oil in a skillet or wok over medium heat. When the oil is heated, stir in your garlic and your ginger and allow them to cook for 1 minute. Add your cubed tofu to your pan of ginger and garlic, pouring in your soy sauce along with the tofu. Stir to coat the tofu in the mixture, and then cover the pan for 25 to 30 minutes, stirring occasionally. Finish off your cooked tofu with a squeeze of fresh lime. You can easily pair your ginger and garlic tofu with some fresh noodles and a little peanut sauce for a quick, Thai-style meal.

Green Gazpacho

2 slices whole-grain bread, crusts removed
3 ripe Hass Avocados, peeled and in chunks
1 green pepper, seeded and chopped
½ cucumber, peeled and chopped
½ medium yellow onion, chopped
2 garlic cloves, chopped

½ cup chopped cilantro
Fresh juice of 1 lemon
½ cup extra virgin olive oil
1 teaspoon cumin
1 pinch of crushed red pepper
1 cup distilled water

Directions:

Tear bread into chunks, place in bowl with water to cover. When water has been absorbed, drain in a colander, press gently to remove excess liquid and set aside.

In a blender, combine avocado, green pepper, cucumber, onion and garlic; blend to smooth consistency. Place mixture into a bowl and set aside. Next, place bread in blender with cilantro and lemon juice and blend till smooth. Slowly add in olive oil. Add the cumin and red pepper until blended. Take all mixtures and blend together. If mixture is too thick, stir in some distilled water to thin.

Egyptian Lentil Soup

\

1 coarsely chopped onion
1 carrot, peeled and chopped
2 ounces of lean Lamb
2 tablespoons extra virgin olive oil
1 tablespoon ground cumin

1 teaspoon ground fennel seeds
1 ½ cups brown lentils
2 quarts distilled water
1 small dried red chili pepper
Juice of 1 lemon

Directions:

In a stockpot or crockpot, gently sauté the onion, carrot, and lamb in olive oil until vegetables are soft and meat is browned. Stir in cumin and fennel and add lentils and distilled water. Add the whole chili pepper and cook until lentils are soft.

When lentils are tender, remove chili pepper. Add lemon juice and stir gently.

Garlic Soup

6 whole heads of garlic cloves, peeled
½ cup extra virgin olive oil
1 tablespoon dried red chili pepper
5 cups chicken stock

½ cup Spanish Sherry
1 pinch of ground cumin
1 pinch of saffron

Directions:

In a soup pot, gently cook garlic in olive oil on low heat until cloves are softened for 10 minutes. Remove with a spoon and set aside. Stir in red chili pepper, then add stock and sherry. Bring to a simmer, while stirring in cumin and saffron.

Use a fork to crush the tender garlic cloves and stir into the soup. Cover and allow soup to simmer, about 15 minutes. Serve with a thick whole-grain bread.

Fish Soup & Wild Rice

2 cups distilled water
1 quart fish stock
2 bay leaves
1 teaspoon dried oregano
1 teaspoon ground black pepper
1 dried chili pepper
1 large onion, coarsely chopped

1 carrot, peeled and coarsely chopped
2 ripe medium tomatoes, quartered
2 pounds of haddock, halibut or cod
2 tablespoons extra virgin olive oil
1 large potato, peeled and cut into bite-sized pieces

Directions:
Combine stock and water in a soup pot; add bay leaf, oregano, pepper, chili, onion, carrot and tomatoes. Bring to a boil and cook over medium low heat until vegetables are very soft. Strain stock.
Return strained stock to the pan and add the fish. Cook at a slow simmer and depending upon thickness, remove from heat after about 20 minutes. Add potato to the stock and cook until tender. Drizzle olive oil over top.

Pasta Checca

6 large ripe, red tomatoes
1 garlic clove, minced
2 medium red onions, thinly sliced
1 cup loosely packed basil leaves

1 tablespoon black pepper
½ cup extra virgin olive oil
3 cups fusilli pasta
2 quarts distilled water

Directions:
In a large bowl, cut tomatoes, garlic and onion. Add basil leaves to bowl, a teaspoon of pepper and olive oil. Cover bowl, set in fridge to marinate. Cook pasta in boiling water; remove bowl from fridge and as soon as pasta is cooked, drain and add pasta to bowl, mixing thoroughly.

Roasted Comforting Vegetables

1 red bell pepper, seeded and sliced

1 green bell pepper, seeded and sliced

1 sweet potato, peeled and cubed

1 bag baby carrots

1 cup mushrooms

3 Russet potatoes, cubed (peeled or not up to you)

1 red onion, coarsely chopped

1 tablespoon chopped fresh thyme

2 tablespoons chopped fresh rosemary

1/2 cup extra virgin olive oil

2 tablespoons lemon juice

1 tablespoon salt

1 tablespoon ground black pepper

Directions:

Preheat oven to 350F degrees. In a large bowl, combine the green and red bell peppers, carrots, sweet potato, red onion and Russet potatoes. Blend all the seasoning ingredients together - rosemary, olive oil, thyme, lemon juice, salt, and pepper. Sprinkle over vegetables and toss to blend thoroughly with vegetables, ensuring all are coated. Place vegetables evenly in a shallow baking dish or roasting pan and bake slowly for 45 minutes, stirring and basting every 15 minutes; before removing from oven, make sure vegetables are thoroughly cooked and tender.

Chakchouka – Moroccan Cooked Tomatoes & Peppers

4 large tomatoes, peeled and seeded, cut into chunks
2 garlic cloves
½ cup extra virgin olive oil

4 sweet peppers
1 green chili pepper
1 tablespoon paprika
1 tablespoon parsley

Directions:
In a skillet cook tomatoes with garlic in olive oil over a medium heat. Stir frequently until tomatoes are cooked down to thick sauce. Cut peppers and chili into pieces and stir into tomatoes. Add paprika and parsley and blend well. Serve with thick breading.

Sweet Crumbed Chicken

2 cups cornflakes, ground
1 cup grated Parmesan cheese
¾ cup plain yogurt

2 tablespoons garlic cloves, minced
4 boneless skinless chicken breasts

Directions:
Preheat oven to 350 degrees. Lightly spray a baking dish with olive oil cooking spray. Mix together the cornflakes and cheese. Coat chicken in yogurt and minced garlic, then dip into the cornflake and cheese mixture; repeat on other side. Bake for 20 minutes or until cooked thoroughly.

Shrimp & Okra Gumbo

2 slices turkey bacon, chopped
½ pound fresh okra, cut into quarters
1 can diced tomatoes

½ chopped yellow onion
1 tablespoon garlic, minced
8 large shrimp, peeled and deveined

Directions:
In a large skillet, sauté turkey bacon until browned. Add fresh okra in the skillet and stir; next add tomatoes. Cook over low heat until okra slightly tender. Add shrimp and continue to cook until shrimp and okra are fully cooked.

Fast Mango Fish

2 pieces of swordfish or mahi mahi
1 cup olive oil

1 tablespoon ground black pepper
2 mangoes, sliced

Directions:
Coat fish liberally with olive oil and black pepper. Heat a non stick skillet over medium heat with ½ cup olive oil. Pan fry fish, flipping sides until cooked. Serve with fresh mango slices.

Beef Massaman Curry

1 pound lean beef strips
1 tablespoon curry paste
1 can (14 ounces) coconut milk

3 red-skinned potatoes, peeled and cubed
½ cup distilled water

Directions:
Place beef strips and ½ cup distilled water in skillet. Cook over high heat until browned. Combine curry paste and coconut milk and add to beef. Add potatoes and turn heat down to low and simmer for 30 minutes or until potatoes are cooked. Serve over brown rice.

Sour-Creamed Meatballs

1 ½ pound extra lean ground beef
1 cup sour cream

1 teaspoon garlic, minced
2 tablespoons olive oil

Directions:
Combine beef, sour cream and garlic and roll into small-sized meatballs. Heat olive oil in a nonstick skillet. Drop in meatballs and fry for 15 minutes over medium heat, until browned on all sides. Place the meatballs on paper towels to drain off excess oil before serving.

Chicken in Tempura Batter

2 tablespoons garlic cloves, minced
2 boneless skinless chicken breasts cut into thin slices
2/3 cup soy flour
1/3 cup cornstarch
8 ounces club soda
1/3 cup olive oil

Directions:
Combine soy flour and cornstarch into a bowl. Make a well in the center and add seltzer, mixing well until smooth and without any lumps. Set aside for about 15 minutes before using. Heat non stick skillet with oil on medium heat. Take sliced chicken breasts, dip each piece into Tempura batter and then place into heated skillet. Allow to fry and brown on each side, until chicken is thoroughly cooked, about 15 minutes.

Fried Green Garlic Tomatoes

1 cup cornmeal
½ cup grated Parmesan cheese
1 tablespoon garlic, minced

4 large green tomatoes cut into thick slices
¼ cup olive oil

Directions:
Mix together the cornmeal and grated parmesan cheese. Coat tomatoes in cornmeal mix, then top with some garlic. In a large nonstick skillet, heat oil over medium heat. Add tomatoes and cook until golden brown on each side, about 3 to 4 minutes.

Zucchini & Veggie Hash Browns

1 cup grated zucchini
2 garlic cloves, minced
1 green bell pepper, diced
2 organic eggs

3 tablespoons olive oil
½ yellow onion
1 tablespoon basil
1 tablespoon rosemary

Directions:
In a medium bowl, mix zucchini, onion, bell pepper, garlic, eggs, basil and rosemary. Heat olive oil in a skillet and gently drop zucchini mixture into hot oil. When browned, turn to other side and brown. Stack on a plate with paper towels.

Easy Broccoli and Cauliflower With Cheese Sauce

1 cup cauliflower
1 cup broccoli
1/4 cup unsalted butter
1/4 cup soy flour
2 cups soy milk
2 cups cheddar cheese
1 dash Worcestershire sauce
salt and pepper to taste

Directions:

Chop the cauliflower and broccoli into medium-sized florets. Steam the florets until they are tender. In a saucepan, melt the butter over medium heat. Sprinkle the soy flour in the pan and slowly add the soy milk, whisking it until it becomes thick and smooth. Add the grated cheese, and Worcestershire sauce;
continue to stir until it is melted and well blended. Add salt and pepper to taste and pour over the steamed vegetables.

Quinoa Soup with Avocado and Corn

4 cups vegetable broth
1 cup quinoa flakes
1 cup frozen corn

¼ cup chunky salsa
1 ripe Avocado, diced
3 tablespoons fresh cilantro

Directions:
In a large soup pot, bring vegetable broth to a boil over high heat. Slowly stir in the quinoa flakes; boil for about 4 to 5 minutes. Stir in corn and salsa and continue cooking until soup is thick, about 2 minutes. Remove from heat, stir in the avocado and add salt and cilantro to taste.

Bulgur Salad topped with Tuna, Olives and Feta

3 tablespoons extra virgin olive oil
½ teaspoon oregano
Pinch of salt
1 ¼ coarse bulgur
6 ounces feta cheese
1 can tuna packed in oil

2 ½ cups diced seeded cucumbers
½ cup pitted Kalamata olives, halved
Grated zest of 1 lemon
¼ cup freshly squeezed lemon juice
Black pepper to taste
3 cups distilled water

Directions:
Pour olive oil into small bowl. Sprinkle oregano in oil and stir, set aside. In a heavy 2-quart pot, bring 3 cups distilled water to a boil and slowly add the bulgur. Stir and cover and allow to simmer, until grains are tender, about 20 minutes. Drain. Run under cold water to cool. Crumble feta into a salad bowl. Add tuna, cucumbers, olives and bulgur. Toss in the olive oil-oregano mixture and add lemon zest and juice.

Wild Rice and Turkey Salad w/ fruit

1 ¼ cups instant wild rice
½ teaspoon salt
2 ½ cups diced, cooked roasted turkey
2 navel oranges, peeled and separated into segments
1 Granny Smith apple, diced
¼ cup dried cranberries
½ cup hazelnuts, coarsely chopped
3 tablespoons mayonnaise
½ cup orange juice
1 ¼ cup distilled water

Directions:
Combine rice and 1 ¼ cups distilled water in a deep pot. Bring to a boil over high heat. Cover and reduce heat and let simmer. Cook for 5 minutes, stir well then remove from heat and set aside. Combine turkey, oranges, apple, cranberries and hazelnuts in a bowl. In a separate bowl, blend mayonnaise and orange juice. When rice is done, drain and toss in salad. Stir in dressing and add salt.

Smoked Trout with yogurt dressed Pasta

8 ounces whole-grain ziti
1 cup low-fat yogurt
2 tablespoons horseradish
2 tablespoons chopped capers
6 ounces smoked trout

2 cups cherry tomatoes
1/3 cup parsley
6 cups shredded Romaine
2 cups distilled water

Directions:
Bring a pot of distilled water to a boil, add the pasta and cook according to package. While pasta is boiling you can prepare the yogurt sauce. In large bowl, blend yogurt, horseradish and capers; add the smoked trout to yogurt mixture.
When pasta is done and drained, toss pasta, tomatoes and parsley into the yogurt sauce. Gently toss with Romaine.

Snacks

True Blue Smoothie

1 medium very ripe banana, broken into chunks
1 cup frozen blueberries

1/2 to 1 cup unflavored or vanilla milk or alternative of choice (almond milk, coconut milk beverage, and rice milk)
1/4 cup packed fresh baby spinach leaves
1/2 cup ice

Directions:
Place ripe banana, blueberries, and 1/2 cup of milk into your blender, and process until smooth. Add in the baby spinach leaves and continue to blend.

Banana Nut Milkshake

1 frozen banana, slice into mid-sized chunks
1 tablespoon peanut butter, creamy
1/2 cup unsweetened almond milk

½ teaspoon vanilla extract
chopped almonds for garnish

Directions:
Blend all ingredients in a blender on high until smooth. Garnish with almonds as desired and serve.

Choco Smoothie

1 large, very ripe banana sliced into mid-sized chunks and frozen
   1 ½ cups unsweetened chocolate soy milk

1/2 ounce slivered almonds
1 to 2 teaspoons cocoa powder
½ teaspoon cinnamon

Directions:
Remove frozen banana from freezer and combine with 3/4 cup of the soy milk in your blender; mix gently. Add more soy milk as needed to get the consistency you want. Blend in the almonds, and tablespoons of cocoa powder. Sprinkle with cinnamon.

Tropical Smoothie

1 peach, cut into chunks
1 mango, cut into chunks
1/2 cup coconut milk

1/2 cup orange juice
1-2 tablespoon coconut flakes

Directions: Blend until smooth and creamy.

Beach Blonde Smoothie

1 banana, peeled & broken in chunks
1 white nectarine pitted and chopped or a peach can be substituted
1/2 cup fresh or frozen pineapple chunks

2 tablespoons almond butter
3/4 cup rice milk or almond milk
1/4 teaspoon vanilla extract
1 tablespoon ground flax seed

Directions: Place all ingredients in blender and mix well.

Mango Lime Smoothie

2 cups frozen mango chunks
1 cup non-dairy milk of choice

1 tablespoon lime juice

Directions: Place all ingredients in your blender and mix until smooth and creamy.

Pumpkin Protein Smoothie

1/3 cup canned pumpkin, chilled
1/2 banana, frozen
3/4 cup vanilla soy milk or almond milk
1 teaspoon maple syrup

3/4 to 1 scoop whey protein powder, vanilla
1/2 teaspoon pumpkin spice
1/4 teaspoon ground cinnamon

Directions: Mix all ingredients in a blender until smooth and creamy.

Homemade Granola with Yogurt

6 cups oats
2 cups nuts/seeds (almonds, pecans, sesame)
2 cups dried cranberries
1/2 cup (or more) flax meal
1/2 cup agave nectar or raw honey
1 cup canned pumpkin
4-6 peeled and grated apples, or 1/2 cup nut or seed butter
2 tablespoons olive oil
Spice mixture (2 teaspoons cinnamon, 1 teaspoon nutmeg, 1/2 teaspoon ground ginger)
Unflavored yogurt

Directions:
Preheat oven to 300°F. Mix all the ingredients and place in a baking dish. Mix it up well to be sure that all oats and nuts are coated in the oil and sweetener, and spread the granola into a single layer. Bake uncovered for 60 minutes, stirring often

Pear & Raspberry Crumble

4 pears, peeled and cut into medium-sized chunks
2 apples, peeled; slice into mid-sized wedges
1 cup fresh or frozen raspberries
1/2 lemon, juiced
1/2 cup whole wheat flour
2 cups old-fashioned rolled oats

3 tablespoons brown sugar
1 teaspoon cinnamon
1 pinch salt
2 tablespoons coconut oil
1/4 cup raw honey
2 tablespoons cornstarch
1/4 cup pecans, chopped
1/4 cup shredded coconut

Directions:
Preheat oven to 450°F. Combine the fruit - pears, apples, raspberries, with the lemon juice, brown sugar, cornstarch, cinnamon, and salt. Spread in a medium baking dish (9×13-inch works well). Melt the margarine and raw honey over medium heat. Remove saucepan from the heat and slowly blend in the flour; blend well so there are no lumps. Blend in the oats, pecans, and shredded coconut. Blend well until oats have become moist and the mixture is crumbly. Take the oat mixture and spread over top the fruit mixture evenly in the baking dish. Top with an additional sprinkle of cinnamon, if desired. Cover with aluminum foil, place in oven for 30 minutes. Remove foil and bake an additional 15 minutes, or until fruit is soft and topping crisps.

Banana Raspberry Soft Serve

1 frozen banana, broken into chunks
1 pinch ground flax seed
½ cup raspberries

1 teaspoon SPLENDA brown sugar
1/4 cup granola

Directions:
Puree your frozen banana with a blender, then mix with ground flaxseed or flaxseed meal. Sprinkle with brown sugar, raspberries, and granola.

Quick Crepes

1/2 cup distilled water
1/2 cup unsweetened almond or coconut milk
1/4 teaspoon salt

3/4 cup whole wheat pastry flour or soy flour
2 tablespoons butter or dairy-free margarine

Directions:
Pour water, milk alternative, and salt into a blender and blend well. Add in whole-wheat or soy flour, then margarine. Blend for about one minute then place in fridge to chill the batter – about 1 hour. Heat up a pan with oil, and using a 1/4 measuring cup, pour in the batter. Swirl the pan so the batter evens out, making a thin pancake. Cook until golden, for about a minute, then turn to other side. Top with whatever you wish.
Stuff with a little reduced fat cream cheese (or dairy-free cream cheese alternative) and some fresh strawberries.

Apricot Balls

¾ cup mixed dried fruit
¼ cup dried apricots

1 tablespoon coconut milk
1 cup shredded coconut

Directions:
Place mixed fruit, apricots and coconut milk in blender on low. Next, shape balls and roll into shredded coconut. Chill in refrigerator until apricot balls become firm.

Sesame Honey Snack Bars

1 cup sesame seeds
1 cup old-fashioned rolled oats

½ cup raw honey
½ cup unsalted butter

Directions:
Preheat oven to 350F. Blend or grind sesame seeds and oats together in blender. Melt honey and butter in a small saucepan, then pour mixture into blender. Mix, place into baking dish, lined with parchment paper. Bake for 20 to 25 minutes, until a toasty golden brown. Cut into snack-size bars.

Sweet Potato Pudding

1 large can sweet potatoes
2 organic eggs, lightly beaten
1 cup packed brown SPLENDA sugar
1 cup almond milk
1/4 cup melted unsalted butter

2 lemons juiced
½ teaspoon ground ginger
½ teaspoon ground cloves
½ teaspoon ground cinnamon
½ teaspoon salt

Directions:
Preheat an oven to 350 degrees F. Slightly spray a baking dish. Combine sweet potatoes and 2 eggs in a bowl and add in the SPLENDA brown sugar, almond milk, butter, lemon juice, ginger, cloves, cinnamon, and salt. Blend ingredients thoroughly then place into prepared dish. Bake until golden brown, about 30 minutes.

Banana Nut Cookies

2 mashed up bananas
2 tablespoons melted coconut oil
½ teaspoon vanilla extract
1/3 cup almond flour
4 tablespoons chopped walnuts

½ teaspoon sea salt
½ teaspoon baking powder
1 cup quinoa flakes
½ teaspoon cinnamon

Directions:

Line a baking tray with parchment paper and preheat oven to 350ºF. Combine bananas with melted coconut oil. In a large mixing bowl combine the quinoa flakes, almond flour, chopped walnuts, sea salt, baking powder and cinnamon. Stir the banana and oil and make into dough. Form into dough balls about 1-1/2 inches in diameter and place on baking tray.

Using the bottom of a glass, flatten each ball to about ½ -inch thickness. Bake cookies for 8-10 minutes, or until lightly browned yet firm. Allow to cool.

Fruit on-a-stick

1/3 cup seedless grapes, red
1/3 cup seedless grapes, green
1 apple
1 banana

½ cup canned pineapple, chunks
1 cup plain yogurt
1/4 cup shredded coconut

Directions:

Wash all fruit and cut into small squares. Peel bananas and cut into chunks. Spread fruit onto a large tray. Spread coconut onto another tray. Place fruit onto the stick – design how you want and place whichever fruit you want. Continue from beginning of stick to end. Hold at each end and roll fruit in the yogurt, and then roll in the coconut. Make sure all fruit is covered.

Nutty Maple Oaties

1/2 cup nut butter
1/2 cup maple syrup or agave nectar
1/2 cup unsweetened shredded coconut
1/2 cup chopped nuts (can substitute seeds for "nut-free")

1/2 cup chocolate/carob chips or dried fruit
1 teaspoon vanilla extract
1 teaspoon ground cinnamon
1/4 to 1/2 teaspoon salt

Directions:

Preheat oven to 325°F. Mix ingredients and place in fridge for about 15 minutes. Scoop cookie dough by the tablespoonful (a melon ball scooper works well) onto a parchment lined or greased cookie sheet. Bake 10-12 minutes. Allow to cool and then form into small balls before placing on the cooling rack.

Berry Choco-Muffins

1 cup pulp-free orange juice
½ cup coconut oil
½ cup SPLENDA brown sugar
1/2 teaspoon salt
2 cups or whole wheat flour (do not get rising)
1 teaspoon baking powder
½ teaspoon baking soda

½ cup semi-sweet chocolate chips
1/4 cup cocoa powder
1/4 teaspoon cinnamon
½ cup rolled oats
½ cup fresh red currants
½ cup frozen or fresh raspberries

Directions:

Lightly grease 12 muffin cups and preheat oven to 350°F. Mix your pulp-free orange juice, coconut oil, SPLENDA brown sugar, and salt. In a separate bowl, sift whole wheat flour, baking powder and baking soda, cocoa, and cinnamon. Stir in the oats. Combine all of your berries and chocolate chips into the dry mixture, and toss together. Take the pulp-free orange juice, coconut oil, SPLENDA brown sugar, and salt and mix with whole wheat flour, baking powder and baking soda, cocoa, berries, chocolate chips and cinnamon; stir carefully so you do not mash the berries. Spoon batter into the muffin cups; Do not fill all the way - about 1/3 inch from the top. Bake for about 20 minutes.

Vanilla Custard

3 organic eggs, lightly beaten
Olive oil cooking spray
1/3 cup SPLENDA sugar
1 teaspoon vanilla extract

2 cups soy milk
1/4 teaspoon ground nutmeg
¼ teaspoon cinnamon

Directions:

Combine eggs, sugar, vanilla extract and soy milk in a mixing bowl; mix well. Lightly spray a baking dish with olive oil cooking spray. Pour mixture into a lightly buttered baking dish; you can also use a soufflé dish which is deeper, and sprinkle with nutmeg and cinnamon.

Old Indian Comfort Pudding

3 cups soy milk
1/2 cup polenta
1/2 teaspoon salt
3 organic eggs
1/4 cup light brown SPLENDA sugar

1/3 cup maple syrup
2 tablespoon unsalted butter
1/2 teaspoon cinnamon
1/4 teaspoon allspice
1/2 teaspoon ginger

Directions:

Lightly spray a soufflé dish with olive oil cooking spray. Preheat oven on 350F. In a saucepan bring soy milk, cornmeal and salt to a boil, stirring constantly, for 5 minutes then cover and simmer an additional 10 minutes. Combine the brown SPLENDA sugar, cinnamon, allspice, ginger and eggs; beat in cornmeal mixture slowly and whisk until smooth. Pour into soufflé dish and bake for 2 to 3 hours

Hot Fruit Compote

1 can pears, drained and rinsed
1 can pineapple chunks, drained and rinsed
1 can peaches, drained and rinsed
1 cup brown SPLENDA sugar

1 teaspoon cinnamon
1/2 stick unsalted butter
1 can cherry pie filling

Directions:

Rinse all canned fruit. Dice fruit into bite-size chunks. Combine the SPLENDA, cinnamon, unsalted butter and the can of cherry pie filling. Stir and mix well. Pour into a medium saucepan, cover and simmer on low heat for about 2 hours.

Ginger Brown Snack Bread

1 package gingerbread mix
1/4 cup polenta
1 teaspoon salt

1-1/2 cups soy milk
1/2 cup golden raisins

Directions:

Preheat oven to 350F. In a medium sized bowl, combine gingerbread mix with polenta and salt; stir in soy milk and then beat with an electric mixer. Next, add the raisins. Grease and flour a loaf pan and pour mixture into it. Bake the snack bread for 1 hour. Top snack bread with cream cheese and serve warm.

Sticky Sugared Nuts

2 cups pecan halves
¼ cup unsalted butter, melted
¼ coconut oil
1/3 cup agave nectar

1 tablespoon cinnamon
1/4 teaspoon ginger
1/4 teaspoon ground allspice

Directions:

Stir the pecans, coconut oil and unsalted butter in a medium sized pot until ingredients are combined. Add agave nectar, stirring to coat. Cover and cook on high for 10 minutes. Turn to low heat and cook uncovered for about 1 hour, or until the nuts are covered with a crisp glaze. Place into a dish and top with cinnamon, ginger and allspice.

Spooned Peaches

1/3 cup SPLENDA brown sugar
2 teaspoon coconut oil
Non stick cooking spray
1/2 cup vanilla flavored soy milk
3/4 cup rice flour

2 organic eggs
2 cups peaches, mashed
2 teaspoon vanilla extract
3/4 teaspoon cinnamon

Directions:

Preheat oven 300F. Spray soufflé dish with non-stick cooking spray. Combine SPLENDA and rice flour. Add organic eggs and vanilla extract. Add coconut oil and milk. Add in cinnamon and mashed peaches. Bake for 1 hour.

Caramel Apples

4 large tart apples, cored
1/2 cup apple juice
4 Tablespoons molasses

4 Tablespoon coconut oil
8 pieces of caramel
1/4 teaspoon ground cinnamon

Directions:

Peel each apple; place in deep baking dish and pour apple juice over apples. Sprinkle the very top of each apple with 2 Tablespoons of molasses and 1 Tablspoon of coconut oil. Place one piece of caramel on the top of each apple and then sprinkle with cinnamon. Place in oven for 1 hour or until apples are tender.

Dessert Recipes

Single Surprise Chocolate Chip Cake

4 tablespoons soy flour (this recipe should not use any self-rising flour)
3 tablespoons SPLENDA or another sugar substitute
2 tablespoons of hot chocolate mix
1/4 teaspoon baking powder

1 organic egg or use egg beaters
3 tablespoons almond or soy milk
2 tablespoons coconut oil
3 tablespoons chocolate chips (optional)
1 tablespoon of vanilla extract

Directions:
Use a coffee mug for single-servings. Add soy flour, sugar, cocoa, and baking powder and mix well. Next, add milk, egg and oil. Add vanilla extract and chocolate chips and mix. Microwave for 2.25 minutes. Remove and allow the dessert to cool.

Love in a Cup - Red Velvet Dessert

3 tablespoons coconut flour

2 tablespoons cocoa powder

1/4 teaspoon baking soda

1 organic egg

2 tablespoons coconut oil

3 tablespoons low fat buttermilk

4 tablespoons SPLENDA or another food substitute

1 tablespoon vanilla extract

5 drops red food coloring

Directions:
Use an oversized cup or coffee mug. Add coconut flour, sugar, cocoa, baking powder and mix well. Next, add low fat buttermilk, egg and coconut oil. Add in the vanilla extract and a few drops of red food coloring and mix. Microwave for 2 minutes 25 seconds. Remove, allow cooling then top with raspberries and vanilla bean ice cream.

Comforting Corn Pudding

1 16 oz. can of creamed corn
1 16 oz. sweet can corn, drained and rinsed
1 cup of sour cream

1/2 cup non-salted butter, melted
1 pkg. cornbread mix

Directions:
In a bowl, mix creamed corn, sweet corn, sour cream and melted unsalted butter. Stir in packaged cornbread mix; blend all well. Coat baking dish with non-stick olive oil spray then pour batter into the dish. Bake, uncovered, at 375 degrees for 30 to 40 minutes,

Coffee-Creamed Brownies

Unsweetened baking chocolate, 3 squares broken up
2 organic eggs, beaten
1 cup SPLENDA sugar
1 tablespoon vanilla extract
½ cup unsalted butter, softened and divided
2/3 cup whole wheat flour, do not use self rising
¼ teaspoon baking soda
1 teaspoon instant coffee
1/3 cup plus 1 tablespoon whipping cream, divided
1 cup semi-sweet chocolate chips

Directions:
Over low heat, melt baking chocolate and ½ cup unsalted butter; allow to cool. Whisk eggs, SPLENDA and vanilla extract. Stir in melted chocolate. Combine whole wheat flour and baking soda; add to the chocolate mixture. Grease a long baking dish, pour mixture into it. Bake at 350 degrees for 25 to 30 minutes. Allow to cool. In a separate bowl, stir in instant coffee into one of whipping tablespoon cream cups; stir until dissolved. Whisk in the remaining SPLENDA sugar and unsalted butter until creamy; spread over brownies. In a small pan begin to melt chocolate chips and the remaining whipped cream over low heat, until it thickens. Spread mixture over layer of cream. Allow to completely cool and cut into squares.

Mediterranean Citrus & Olive Oil Cake

1 orange
1 lemon
3 cups cake flour
1 teaspoon baking soda
1 tablespoon cinnamon

2 ½ cups of currants
1 cup extra virgin olive oil
1 ½ cups SPLENDA sugar
1 tablespoon brandy extract

Directions:
Preheat oven at 350F degrees and spray cake pan with olive oil cooking spray and set aside. Grate the zest of an orange and lemon and mix. Squeeze the orange and lemon juice and mix with the zest.
Sift flour with the baking soda and cinnamon. Add currants, stirring to distribute evenly through flour. In medium sized bowl add sugar and oil and beat. Add mixtures together. Finally, add the brandy extract and mix well. Pour batter into greased pan and bake for 1 hour. Remove and let cool.

Berry Cake

1 ½ cup raspberries
1 ½ cup blueberries
5 beaten organic eggs
1 2/3 cup SPLENDA sugar

1-1/4 cup unsalted butter, diced and softened
2 tablespoon blackberry syrup
1 teaspoon baking powder
2-1/2 cup soy flour

Directions:
Combine the eggs and SPLENDA in a bowl and set aside. In a separate bowl, whisk butter and blackberry syrup and blend well. Add the sugar/butter mixture to the eggs; stir in baking powder. Blend well and set aside. Next, in a separate bowl, combine all berries and the remaining soy flour; blend well. Gently combine all ingredients into one bowl. Prepare a Bundt cake pan by greasing and flour; pour mixture into pan and place in oven at 325 degrees; bake for about one hour or until completely done.

Apple Crock Pot Betty

3 lb. cooking apples
Whole grain bread, 5 slices. cubed (about 4 cups)
1/2 teaspoon cinnamon

1/4 teaspoon nutmeg
1/8 teaspoon salt
3/4 cup SPLENDA brown sugar
1/2 cup unsalted butter, melted

Directions:
Thoroughly clean apples and peel. Slice and line them in bottom of crock pot. Combine the cinnamon, nutmeg, salt, SPLENDA, and unsalted butter; blend together. Mix with bread cubes. Pour mixture on top of apples and cover. Cook on low setting for about 2 to 4 hours.

Soft Carrot Pudding

4 carrots, washed
1 small onion, grated
1/4 teaspoon nutmeg

1 tablespoon SPLENDA sugar
1 cup soy milk
3 organic eggs, beaten

Directions:
Wash and grate carrots. Place into small saucepan, cover with water and cook on medium heat until tender. Mash carrots and mix with grated onion, nutmeg, SPLENDA sugar, soy milk, and eggs. Pour into crock pot and cook on high for 3-4 hours.

Banana Nut Cake

½ cup of smashed bananas
1 box of yellow colored cake mix
1 large package of butter pecan instant-pudding mix

4 organic eggs
1 cup distilled water
¼ cup of coconut oil
½ cup of pecans (chopped)

Directions:
Preheat Oven To 350 Degrees. Blend all of the ingredients together in a large mixing bowl until well mixed and you have formed a thick cake batter. Pour your banana cake batter into a greased or non-stick baking pan of your choice. Bake at 350 Degrees for 50 minutes. Remove from oven and let cool for 15 minutes.

Banana Spice Cake

2 smashed bananas
5 large eggs
2 cups of almond flour
1 teaspoon of baking powder

1 teaspoon of cinnamon
¼ Tablespoon cloves
2 teaspoons of banana extract
1 teaspoon of vanilla extract

Directions:
Preheat oven to 350 degrees. In a large mixing bowl blend your butter, sugar, and cream cheese together. Next add your eggs to the mixture one at a time, making sure to mix well after each egg is added. Next mix your almond flour, baking powder and spices, then add them to the mixture. Add your crushed bananas, banana extracts and vanilla extracts, then mix well one last time. Pour your banana cake batter into a 9 inch greased round cake pan.

Raspberry Pudding Cake

½ oz. of yellow cake mix
½ oz. of instant berry pudding mix
4 large eggs

¼ cup coconut oil
1 cup of fresh raspberries

Directions:
Preheat oven to 350 degrees. In a large mixing bowl blend together cake mix, pudding mix, eggs, water, coconut oil and raspberries until well blended. Pour your berry cake batter in a greased or non-stick 9" round baking pan.
Bake at 350 Degrees for 50-55 minutes or until cake tests done. Remove from oven and allow to cool for 10-15 minutes.

Apple-berry Yogurt Parfait

1 small apple (any variety)
1/4 cup berries (strawberries and blueberries make a great combination)
1 8 ounce container sugar-free yogurt (plain or vanilla)
1/4 cup Kashi Go Lean cereal (All Bran or Oat)
1 packet Splenda (optional)

Directions:

Chop apple and berries into bite-sized pieces. In mixing bowl combine the fruits and cereal. Sprinkle in the packet of Splenda over the fruit mixture. Spoon small amount of yogurt into bottom of glass. Spoon in a layer of the fruit and cereal mixture. Follow with a layer of yogurt and continue until parfait glass is full.

Peanut Butter Candy Log

1/4 cup oats
1/4 cup powdered milk
1/4 cup peanut butter
1/2 teaspoon vanilla
4 packets Splenda
2 teaspoons water
wax paper

Directions:

Mix all ingredients in bowl until blended. You may need to add more water based on your peanut butter consistency. Lay out a piece of wax paper on the counter. Shape mixture into a log on wax paper. Roll the wax paper around the log and twist the ends. Refrigerate to desired firmness. Cut to desired size and serve.

Fabulous Fudge

2 packages cream cheese (8 oz each), softened
1/2 cup chopped pecans or walnuts
2 squares unsweetened chocolate , melted
24 packets Splenda
1 teaspoon vanilla

Directions:

In mixing bowl, add cream cheese, chocolate, Splenda, and vanilla. Beat until smooth. Add in nuts and stir. Pour into a square baking pan and cover with foil. Refrigerate overnight. Remove from refrigerator and cut into equal pieces.

Banana Milkshake

3/4 cup skim milk
3/4 cup vanilla ice cream (or favorite variety)
1 large ripe banana (quartered)
4 packets Splenda
1/8 teaspoon vanilla extract

Directions:

Combine all ingredients in a blender. Blend on a low speed until smooth. This recipe yields two servings. Try chocolate ice cream for a completely different milkshake. Add in 2 tablespoons peanut butter for extra protein and flavor. With the chocolate variety try adding a handful of strawberries.

Cream Puffs

1 package cream cheese (8 ounce), softened
1 package sugar free vanilla instant pudding
(1.4 ounce)
1 egg
6 packets Splenda
1 teaspoon vanilla
olive oil cooking spray

Directions:

Preheat your oven to 350 degrees. Thoroughly spray baking sheet with favorite cooking spray. In mixing bowl, combine cream cheese, pudding, Splenda, egg, and vanilla. Blend until ingredients are incorporated together well. Spoon dough onto cookie sheet, leaving room in between each cookie. Bake 14 to 16 minutes and allow to cool before removing cookies from pan.

Quick Pineapple Orange Gelatin Dessert

1 container of cottage cheese (16 ounce)
1 package sugar free gelatin (3.4 ounce)
1 tub sugar free Cool Whip
1/4 cup crushed pineapple

1/4 cup Mandarin oranges

Directions:

In large bowl, combine cottage cheese and gelatin; spoon in sugar free cool whip, then gently spoon in the pineapples. Chill and serve. Try lemon, orange, apricot, and strawberry gelatin mixes. Other fruits add in well to this also. Try grapes, cherries, and mandarin oranges. This doubles as a wonderful fruit dip.

Apple Pudding Muffins

1 tablespoon baking powder
2 cups whole wheat flour
1/2 teaspoon salt
3/4 cup skim milk
1 teaspoon ground cinnamon
2 egg whites
6 packets Splenda

1 packet vanilla pudding mix
1/4 cup vegetable oil
1 cup chopped apples

Directions:

Preheat oven to 375 degrees. Spray one muffin tin with cooking spray. Beat the egg whites. In separate medium bowl, mix pudding mix, baking powder, flour, salt, and cinnamon. Add in apples to the mixture and gently stir. In another bowl, mix milk and vegetable oil; add in the egg whites. Blend the wet ingredients with the dry ingredients and stir. Do not fill muffin tins completely to top. Bake 20 minutes or until lightly browned.

Orange Dream Mousse

1 package cream cheese (8 ounce), softened
1 cup heavy cream
1 package sugar free orange gelatin (1.4 ounce)
several drops of orange extract
6 ice cubes
sugar free Cool Whip

Directions:

Beat cream cheese until smooth. Add gelatin package to 1 cup boiling water and stir until gelatin is dissolved. Stir in a few drops of orange extract. Add ice cubes to gelatin to cool quickly. Add cooled gelatin to cream cheese and whip until well blended. Add cream. Whip approximately 4 minutes to add air into mixture. Spray gelatin mold with cooking spray then pour in mixture. Refrigerate until set. Serve with Cool Whip.

Lovely Lemon Sorbet

1 lemon peel (diced finely) save 6 zest strips for garnish
12 packets Splenda (or 1/2 cup granulated)
1 cup water
1/2 cup lemon juice
1/2 cup carbonated mineral water

Directions:

In saucepan, stir together diced lemon peel, water, and Splenda. Bring to a boil. Reduce heat and simmer for 5 minutes. Cool. In a pitcher, pour in cooled lemon syrup. Stir in the lemon juice and mineral water and then pour into an ice cream maker and set to make ice cream. Garnish dish with lemon zest.

After Dinner Fruit & Dip

16 ounces vanilla sugar free yogurt
2 packets Swiss Miss sugar free hot cocoa mix
1/2 cup strawberries
1 apple
1 peach
handful of white grapes
1/2 cup cherries
coconut chunks

Directions:

Add yogurt and hot cocoa mix to bowl. Stir until well blended. Chill. While chilling dip, prepare all the fruits. Peel, slice, and dice as needed. Serve pieces on a large plate. Substitute other fresh fruits if these are unavailable. Remove dip from refrigerator and enjoy. Have toothpicks or party appetizer spears available for dipping.

Pear and Apple Compote

4 medium pears (Bartlett or Bosc)
8 medium apples (good cooking variety)
1 ounce water
cinnamon (optional)
6 packets Splenda (optional)

Directions:

Start with the pears and apples peeled. Core and slice into bite sized chunks. Add water to saucepan. Add pears and apples to saucepan. Cook until both fruits are tender. Add fruit to a blender, leaving out 1/3 of the fruit mixture. Blend until smooth. Add blended fruit to fruit chunk mixture and stir. Separate into serving bowls. Sprinkle a packet of Splenda and cinnamon as desired with each serving.

Coconut Almond Macaroons

1 angel food cake mix
1/2 cup water
1 1/2 teaspoons almond extract
2 cups shredded coconut

Directions:

Preheat oven to 350 degrees. In large bowl, combine cake mix, water, and almond extract. Beat on low for 30 seconds. Scrape bowl. Beat on medium for 1 minute then stir coconut into mix. Drop spoonful's of mixture onto baking sheet and place in oven for 10 to 12 minutes or until lightly browned. Transfer paper and cookies to wire racks to cool.

Natural Peanut Butter Cookies

1 cup natural peanut butter
1/2 cup grapeseed oil
½ cup pure maple syrup
2 eggs
2 tablespoon vanilla extract
2 cups soy flour
2/3 cup baking cocoa
2 teaspoons baking soda
1/4 teaspoon salt
1 cup grated chocolate bar
½ cup cranapples - chopped

Directions:

Combine the grapeseed oil, vanilla extract, soy flour, maple syrup, eggs, cocoa and baking soda. Blend well and then add the chocolate and cranapples. Drop by teaspoon full to a preheated cookie sheet. Bake for 8 to 10 minutes until golden brown in a 350 degree oven. These store great in air-tight containers for up to two weeks.

Fruit Parfait Delight

Fresh oranges, cut up
Fresh grapefruit, cut up
Fresh strawberries, cut up
Chopped Almonds
2 of your favorite granola bars, cut up
Cool whip, Lite
Chocolate morsels

Directions:

Alternate fruits, nuts, fiber bars, and cool whip. End with a few chocolate morsels.

Use alternate things, such as kiwi, pineapple, and bananas for the fruits; crushed vanilla and chocolate sugar free cookies; and yogurt for the cool whip. Other morsels are peanut butter or butterscotch, or use sugar free hot fudge chocolate or chocolate sprinkles for the top.

About Minute Help Press

Minute Help Press is building a library of books for people with only minutes to spare. Follow @minutehelp on Twitter to receive the latest information about free and paid publications from Minute Help Press, or visit minutehelp.com.

Cover Image - © mangostock - Fotolia.com

Made in the USA
Columbia, SC
03 January 2019